Virtual Clinical Excursions
for
Potter & Perry:
FUNDAMENTALS OF NURSING, 5th Edition

Virtual Clinical Excursions

for

Potter & Perry:
FUNDAMENTALS OF NURSING, 5th Edition

prepared by

Patricia A. Potter, RN, MSN, PhD (cand.), CMAC Research Scientist

Virtual Clinical Excursions CD-ROM prepared by

Jay Shiro Tashiro, PhD, RN
Director of Systems Design
Wolfsong Informatics
Sedona, Arizona

Gina Long, RN, DNSc
Assistant Professor, Department of Nursing
College of Health Professions
Northern Arizona University
Flagstaff, Arizona

Ellen Sullins, PhD
Director of Research
Wolfsong Informatics
Sedona, Arizona

Michael Kelly, MS
Director of the Center for Research and
Evaluation of Advanced Technologies
in Education
Northern Arizona University
Flagstaff, Arizona

The development of Virtual Clinical Excursions Volume 1 was partially funded by the
National Science Foundation, under grant DUE 9950613.
Principal investigators were Tashiro, Sullins, Long, and Kelly.

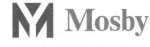

A Harcourt Health Sciences Company

St. Louis   London   Philadelphia   Sydney   Toronto

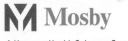

Mosby

A Harcourt Health Sciences Company

Vice President and Publishing Director, Nursing: Sally Schrefer
Executive Editor: June Thompson
Managing Editor: Michele Trope
Project Manager: Gayle Morris
Designer: Wordbench
Cover Art: Kathi Gosche

Mosby, Inc.
A Harcourt Health Sciences Company
11830 Westline Industrial Drive
St. Louis, Missouri 63146

Printed in the United States of America

International Standard Book Number: 0-323-01741-x

01 02 03 04 05 WB/EB 9 8 7 6 5 4 3 2 1

Workbook
prepared by

Patricia A. Potter, RN, MSN, PhD (cand.), CMAC Research Scientist
Barnes-Jewish Hospital
St. Louis, Missouri

Textbook

Patricia A. Potter, RN, MSN, PhD (cand.), CMAC Research Scientist
Barnes-Jewish Hospital
St. Louis, Missouri

Anne Griffin Perry, RN, MSN, EdD
Professor and Co-Coordinator, Adult Health Specialty
Saint Louis University School of Nursing
Saint Louis University Health Sciences Center
St. Louis, Missouri

Contents

Getting Started

Part I—Application of Nursing Concepts

Part II—Caring for Patient's Basic Needs

Part III—Psychosocial Care in Practice

Getting Started

GETTING SET UP

■ MINIMUM SYSTEM REQUIREMENTS

Virtual Clinical Excursions is a hybrid CD, so it runs on both Macintosh and Windows platforms. To use *Virtual Clinical Excursions*, you will need one of the following systems:

- **Windows™**

  Windows 2000, 95, 98, NT 4.0
  IBM compatible computer
  Pentium II processor (or equivalent)
  300 MHz
  96 MB
  800 × 600 screen size
  256 color monitor
  100 MB hard drive space
  12× CD-ROM drive
  Soundblaster 16 soundcard compatibility
  Stereo speakers or headphones

- **Macintosh®**

  MAC OS 9.04
  Apple Power PC G3
  300 MHz
  96 MB
  800 × 600 screen size
  256 color monitor
  100 MB hard drive space
  12× CD-ROM drive
  Stereo speakers or headphones

Ideally, the system you use should have at least 200 MB of free disk space on your hard drive. There are commercially available desktop utility programs that can help clean up your hard drive. No other applications besides the operating system should be running at the time *Virtual Clinical Excursions* is running.

1

■ INSTALLING *VIRTUAL CLINICAL EXCURSIONS*

Virtual Clinical Excursions is designed to run from a set of files on your hard drive and a CD in your CD-ROM. Minimal installation is required.

- **Windows™**

  1. Start Microsoft Windows and insert *Virtual Clinical Excursions* **Disk 1 (Installation)** in the CD-ROM drive.
  2. Click the **Start** icon on the taskbar and select the **Run** option.
  3. Type d:\setup.exe (where "d:\" is your CD-ROM drive) and press OK.
  4. Follow the on-screen instructions for installation.
  5. Remove *Virtual Clinical Excursions* **Disk 1 (Installation)** from your CD-ROM drive.
  6. Restart your computer.

- **Macintosh®**

  1. Insert *Virtual Clinical Excursions* **Disk 1 (Installation)** in the CD-ROM drive. The disk icon will appear on your desktop.
  2. Double-click on the disk icon.
  3. Double-click on the icon **Install Virtual Clinical Excursions**.
  4. Follow the on-screen instructions for installation.
  5. Remove *Virtual Clinical Excursions* **Disk 1 (Installation)** from your CD-ROM drive
  6. Restart your computer.

■ HOW TO RESET YOUR MONITOR TO 256 COLORS

This software will only run if the monitor is set at 256 colors. To reset your monitor:

- **Windows™**

  1. Choose **Settings** from the **Start** menu.
  2. Choose **Control Panel**.
  3. Double-click on the **Display** icon.
  4. Click on the **Settings** tab.
  5. In the **Colors** drop-down menu, click on the arrow to show more settings.
  6. Click on **256 Colors**.
  7. Click on **Apply**.
  8. Click on **OK**.
  9. If the system asks whether you wish to restart your computer to accept these settings, click on **Yes**.

- **Macintosh®**

  1. Choose the **Monitors** control panel.
  2. Change the color display to **256**.

■ **HOW TO USE DISK 2 (PATIENTS' DISK)**

- **Windows™**

    When you want to work with the five patients in the virtual hospital, follow these steps:

    1. Insert *Virtual Clinical Excursions* **Disk 2 (Patients' Disk)** into your CD-ROM drive.
    2. Double-click on the icon **Shortcut to Virtual Clinical Excursions**, which can be found on your desktop. This will load and run the program.

- **Macintosh®**

    When you want to work with the five patients in the virtual hospital, follow these steps:

    1. Insert *Virtual Clinical Excursions* **Disk 2 (Patients' Disk)** into your CD-ROM drive.
    2. Double-click on the icon **Shortcut to Virtual Clinical Excursions**, which can be found on your desktop. This will load and run the program.

■ **QUALITY OF VISUALS, SPEED, AND COMMON PROBLEMS**

Virtual Clinical Excursions uses the Apple QuickTime media layer system. This includes Quick-Time Video and QuickTime VR Video, which allow for high-quality graphics and digital video. The graphics seen in the *Virtual Clinical Excursions* courseware should be of high quality with good color. If the movies and graphics appear blocky or otherwise low-quality, check to see whether your video card is set to "thousands of colors."

Note: Virtual Clinical Excursions is not designed to function at a 256-color depth. (You may need to go to the Control Panel and change the Display settings.) If you don't see any digital video options, please check that QuickTime is installed correctly.

The system should respond quickly and smoothly. In particular, you should not see any jerky motions or unannounced long delays as you move through the virtual hospital settings, interact with patients, or access information resources. If you notice slow, jerky, or delayed software responses, it may mean that your particular system requires additional RAM, your processor does not meet the basic requirements, or your hard drive is full or too fragmented. If the videos appear banded or subject to "breakup," you may need to find an updated video driver for the computer's video card. Please consult the manufacturer of the video card or computer for additional video drivers for your machine.

■ **TECHNICAL SUPPORT**

Technical support for this product is available at no charge by calling the Technical Support Hotline between 9 a.m. and 5 p.m. (Central Time), Monday through Friday. Inside the United States, call 1-800-692-9010. Outside the United States, call 314-872-8370.

A QUICK TOUR

Welcome to *Virtual Clinical Excursions*, a virtual hospital setting in which you can work with five complex patient simulations and also learn to access and evaluate the information resources that are essential for high-quality patient care.

The virtual hospital, Red Rock Canyon Medical Center, is a teaching hospital for Canyonlands State University. Within the medical center, you will work on a medical-surgical floor with a realistic architecture as well as access information resources. The floor plan in which the patient scenarios unfold is constructed from a model of a real medical center. The medical-surgical unit has:

- Five patient rooms (Room 302, Room 303, Room 304, Room 309, Room 310)
- A Nurses' Station (Room 312)
- A Supervisor's Office (Room 301)
- Two conference rooms (Room 307, Room 308)
- A nurses' lounge (Room 306)

■ BEFORE YOU START

Make sure you have your textbook nearby when you use the *Virtual Clinical Excursions Patients' Disk*. You will want to consult topic areas in your textbook frequently while working with the CD and using this workbook.

■ SUPERVISOR'S OFFICE (ROOM 301)

Just like a real-world clinical rotation, you have to let someone know when you arrive on the hospital floor—and you have to let someone know when you leave the floor. This process is completed in the Supervisor's Office (Room 301).

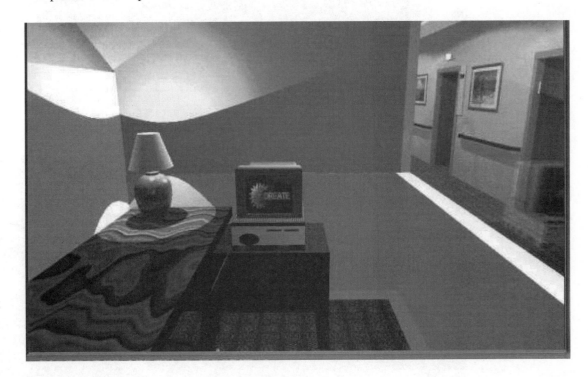

To get a 360° view of where you are "standing":

- Place the cursor in the middle of the screen.
- Hold down the mouse.
- Drag either right or left.

You will see you are in a room with an alcove to your left and a door behind you. To move into the hallway, place the cursor in the door opening and click. Once you are in the hallway, hold down the mouse and make a 360° turn.

In one direction, you will see:

- An exit sign
- An elevator
- A waiting room

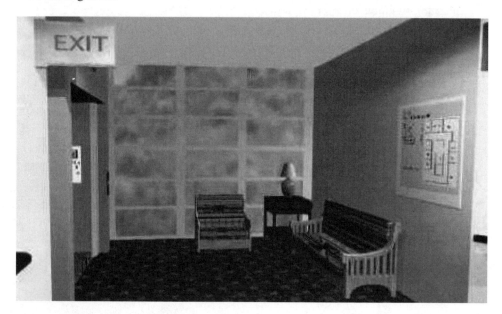

In the other direction, you will see a:

- Patient room
- Mobile computer

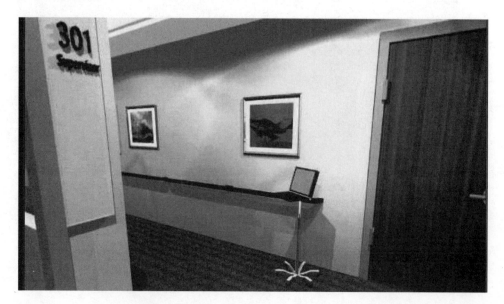

Move the cursor to a new place along the hallway outside the Supervisor's Office and click again. (Always try to place the cursor in the middle of the screen.) You should be moving along the hallway. Remember, at any point you can hold down the mouse and turn 360° in either direction. You can also hold down and move the mouse to the top or bottom of the frame, giving you views looking up or down.

■ READING ROOM

Go back into the Supervisor's Office by clicking on anything inside the room. Explore the Supervisor's Office (Room 301), and you will find another computer. This computer is a link to Canyonlands State University, the simulated university associated with the Red Rock Canyon Medical Center. Double-click on this computer, and a Web browser screen will be launched, which will open the Medical-Nursing Library in Canyonlands State University.

Click on the **Reading Room** icon, and you will see a table of icons that allows you to read short learning modules on a variety of anatomy and physiology topics.

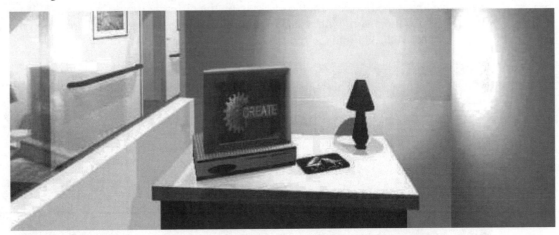

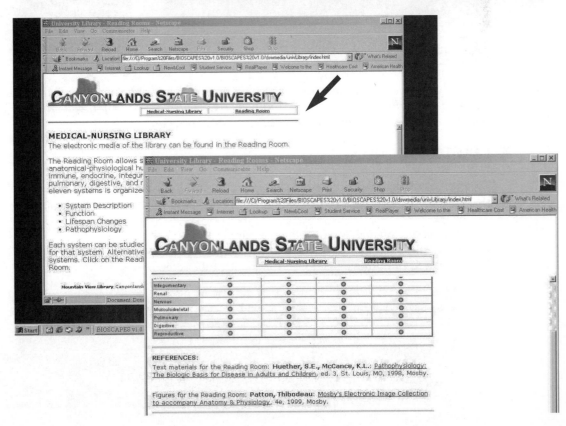

When you are ready to exit the reading room, go to the **File** icon on the browser, look at the drop-down menu, and select **Exit** or **Close**, depending on your Web browser. The browser will close, and once again you will be looking at the computer in the Supervisor's Office.

■ FLOOR MAP AND ANIMATED MAP

Move into the hallway outside the Supervisor's Office and turn right. A floor map can be found on the wall in the waiting area opposite the elevator and exit sign. To get there, click on anything in the waiting area. You should be able to see the map now, but you may not be close enough to open it. Click again on an object in the waiting area; this will move you closer. Turn to the right until you can see the map. Double-click on the map, and you will get a close-up view of the medical-surgical floor's layout. Click on the **Return** icon to exit this close-up view of the floor map.

Compare the floor map on the wall with the animated map in the upper right-hand corner of your screen. The green dot follows your position on the floor to show you where you are. You can move about the floor by double-clicking on the different rooms in this map. If you have already signed in to work with a patient, double-clicking on the patient's room on the animated map will take you right into the room.

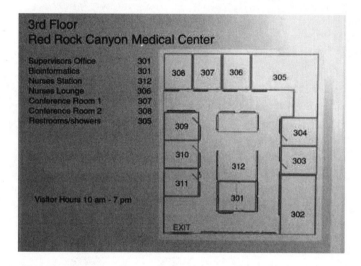

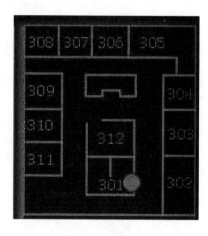

Note: If you have not signed in to work with a patient, double-clicking on a patient's room on the animated map will take you to the hallway right outside the room. If you have not yet selected a patient, you cannot access patient rooms or records.

■ HOW TO SIGN IN

To select a patient, you will need to sign in on the desktop computer in the Supervisor's Office (Room 301). Double-click on the computer screen, and a log-on screen will appear.

- Replace *Student Name* with your name.
- Replace the student ID number with your student ID number.
- Click **Continue** in the lower right side of the screen.

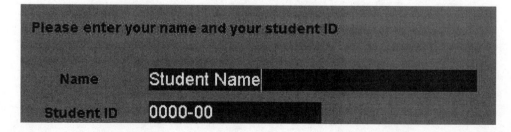

■ HOW TO SELECT A PATIENT

You can choose any one of five patients to work with. For each patient you can select either of two 4-hour shifts on Tuesday or Thursday (0700–1100 or 1100–1500). You can also select a Friday morning period in which you can review all of the data for the patient you selected. You will not, however, be able to visit patients on Friday, only review their records.

■ PATIENT LIST

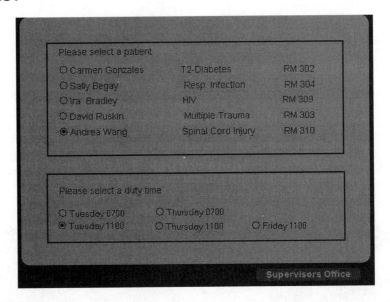

- **Carmen Gonzales (Room 302)**

  Diabetes mellitus, type 2 – An older Hispanic female with an infected leg that has become gangrenous. She has type 2 diabetes mellitus, as well as complications of congestive heart failure and osteomyelitis.

- **David Ruskin (Room 303)**

  Motor vehicle accident – A young adult African-American male admitted with a possible closed head injury and a severely fractured right humerus following a car-bicycle accident. He undergoes an open reduction and internal fixations of the right humerus.

- **Sally Begay (Room 304)**

  Respiratory infection – A Native American woman initially suspected to have a Hantavirus infection. She has a confirmed diagnosis of bacterial lung infection. This patient's complications include chronic obstructive pulmonary disease and inactive tuberculosis.

- **Ira Bradley (Room 309)**

  HIV-AIDS – A Caucasian adult male in late-stage HIV infection admitted for an opportunistic respiratory infection. He has complications of oral fungal infection, malnutrition, and wasting. Patient-family interactions also provide opportunities to explore complex psychosocial problems.

- **Andrea Wang (Room 310)**

  Spinal cord injury – A young Asian female who entered the hospital after a diving accident in which her T6 was crushed, with partial transection of the spinal cord. After a week in ICU, she has been transferred to the Medical-Surgical unit, where she is being closely monitored.

Note: You can select only one patient for one time period. If you are assigned to work with multiple patients, return to the Supervisor's Office to switch from one patient to another.

■ HOW TO FIND A PATIENT'S RECORDS

Nurses' Station (Room 312)

Within the Nurses' Station, you will see:

1. A blue notebook on the counter—this is the Medication Administration Record (MAR).
2. A bookshelf with patient charts.
3. Two desktop computers—the computer to the left of the bulletin board is used to access Red Rock Canyon Medical Center's Intranet; the computer to the right beneath the bookshelf is used to access the Electronic Patient Record (EPR). *(Note: You can also access the EPR from the mobile computer outside the Supervisor's Office, next to Room 302.)*
4. A bulletin board—this contains important information for students.

As you use these resources, you will always be able to return to the Nurses' Station (Room 312) by clicking either a **Nurses' Station** icon or a **3rd Floor** icon located next to the red cross in the lower right-hand corner of the computer screen.

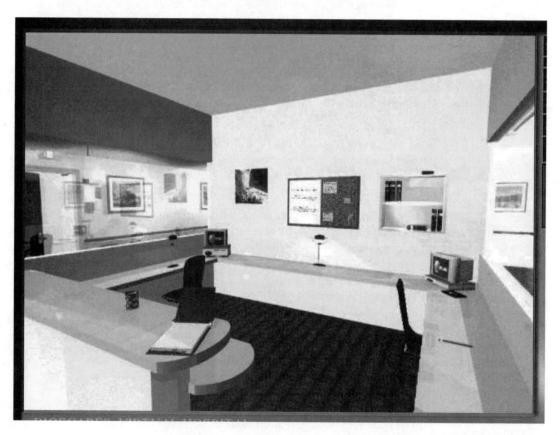

1. Medication Administration Record (MAR)

The blue notebook on the counter in the Nurses' Station (Room 312) is the Medication Administration Record (MAR), listing current 24-hour medications for each patient. Simply click on the MAR, and it opens like a notebook. Tabs allow you to select patients by room number. Each MAR sheet lists the following:

- Medications
- Route and dosage of medications
- Times of administration of medication

The MAR changes each day.

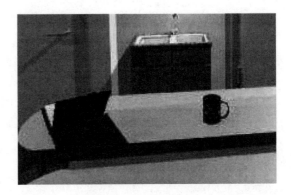

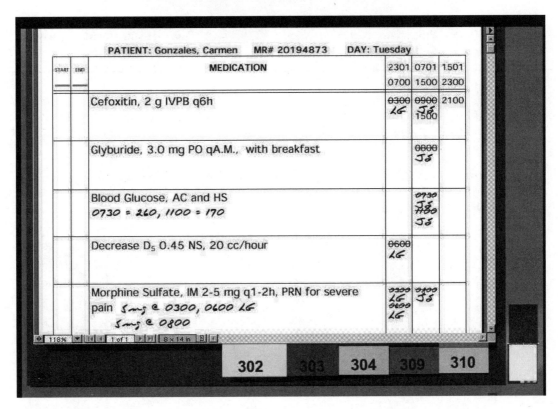

PATIENT: Gonzales, Carmen	MR# 20194873	DAY: Tuesday			
START	END	**MEDICATION**	2301 0700	0701 1500	1501 2300
		Cefoxitin, 2 g IVPB q6h	~~0300~~ *LG*	~~0900~~ *JS* 1500	2100
		Glyburide, 3.0 mg PO qA.M., with breakfast		~~0800~~ *JS*	
		Blood Glucose, AC and HS 0730 = 260, 1100 = 170		~~0730~~ *JS* ~~1100~~ *JS*	
		Decrease D$_5$ 0.45 NS, 20 cc/hour	~~0600~~ *LG*		
		Morphine Sulfate, IM 2-5 mg q1-2h, PRN for severe pain 5mg @ 0300, 0600 LG 5mg @ 0800	~~0300~~ *LG* ~~0600~~ *LG*	~~0800~~ *JS*	

| 302 | 303 | 304 | 309 | 310 |

2. Charts

In the back right-hand corner of the Nurses' Station (Room 312) is a bookshelf with patient charts. To open a chart:

- Double-click on the bookshelf.
- Click once on the chart of your choice.

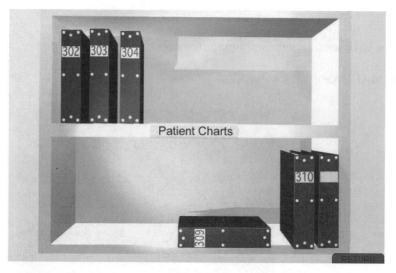

Tabs at the bottom of each patient's chart allow you to review the following data:

- Physical & History*
- Physicians' Notes
- Physicians' Orders
- Nurses' Notes
- Diagnostics Reports

- Expired MARs
- Health Team Reports
- Surgeons' Notes
- Other Reports

"Flip" forward by selecting a tab or backward by clicking on the small chart icon in the lower right side of your screen. (**Flip Back** appears on this icon once you have moved beyond the first tab.) As in the real world, the data in each patient's chart changes daily.

Note: Physical & History is a seven-page PDF file for Carmen Gonzales, David Ruskin, and Ira Bradley. Physical & History is a five-page PDF file for Andrea Wang and Sally Begay. Remember to scroll down to read all pages.

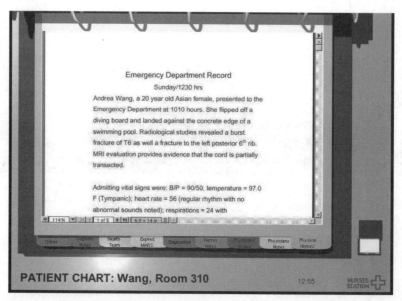

3. Two Computers

◆   **Electronic Patient Record (EPR)**

You can only access an Electronic Patient Record (EPR) once you have signed in and selected the patient in the Supervisor's Office (Room 301). The EPR can be accessed from two computers:

- Desktop computer under the bookshelf in the Nurses' Station (Room 312)
- Mobile computer outside the Supervisor's Office, next to Room 302

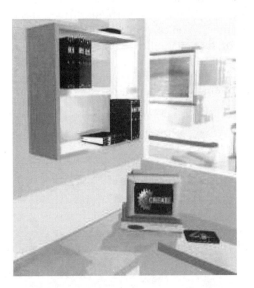
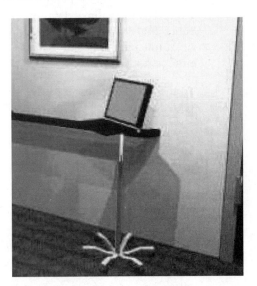

To access a patient's EPR:

- Double-click on the computer screen.
- Type in the password—it will always be **rn2b**.
- Click on **Access Records**.
- Click on the patient's name, then on **Access EPR** (or simply double-click on the patient's name).

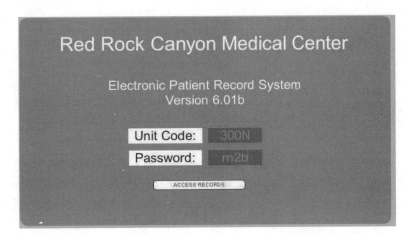

Note: Do **not** *press the Return/Enter key. If you make a mistake, simply delete the password, reenter it, and click* **Access Records**. *You will then enter the records system, where you find a list of patients.*

The EPR form represents a composite of commercial versions being used in hospitals and clinics. You can access the EPR:

- For a patient
- To review existing data
- To enter data you collect while working with a patient

The EPR is updated daily, so no matter what day or part of a shift you are working, there will be a current EPR with the patient's data from the past days of the current hospital stay. This type of simulated EPR allows you to examine how data for different attributes have changed over time, as well as to examine data for all of a patient's attributes at a particular time. The EPR is fully functional (as it is in a real-life hospital or clinic). You can enter such data as blood pressure, heart rate, and temperature. The EPR will not, however, allow you to enter data for a previous time period.

At the lower left corner of the EPR, there are nine icons that allow you to view different types of patient data:

- Assessment
- Admissions
- Urinalysis
- Vital Signs
- ADL

- Blood Gases
- I&O
- Chemistry
- Hematology

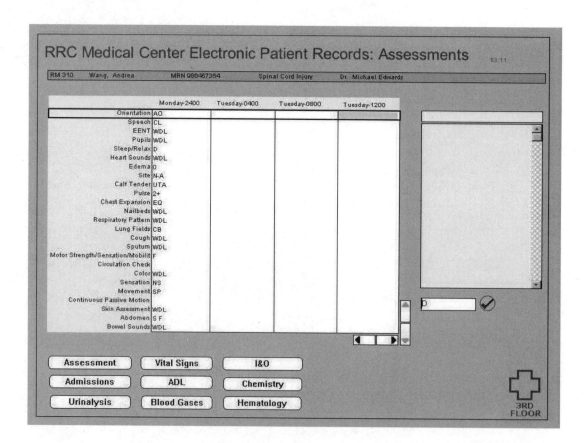

Remember, each hospital or clinic selects its own codes. The codes in the Red Rock Canyon Medical Center may be different from ones you have seen in clinical rotations that have computerized patient records.

You use the codes for the data type, selecting the code to describe your assessment findings and typing that code in the box in the lower right side of the screen, to the left of the checkmark symbol (✓).

Once the data are typed in this box, they are entered into the patient's record by clicking on the checkmark (✓). Make sure you are in the correct cell by looking for the placement of the blue box in the table. That box identifies which cell the database is "looking" at for any given moment.

You can leave the EPR by clicking on the **3rd Floor** icon in the lower right corner. This takes you back into the Nurses' Station (Room 312).

◆ Intranet

The computer on the left of the bulletin board in the Nurses' Station (Room 312) is dedicated to Red Rock Canyon Medical Center's **Intranet**. This system contains resources related to working within the hospital. Again, a double click on the screen will activate the computer. A Web browser will come up with four options (Hospital News, Employment, InfoStat, and Home). Navigate within the Intranet just as you would within a Web-based Internet site. Click on **Hospital News** and read some of the articles. The Employment icon opens a screen with descriptions of jobs available in the hospital. The InfoStat icon will connect the hospital Intranet to the Internet. *(Note: This option searches for your Internet connection, activates that connection, and takes you to the publisher's Website for your textbook.)* When in doubt, click on **Home**, which will take you back to the home page for the site.

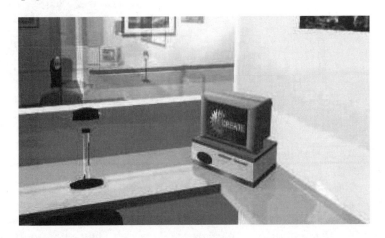

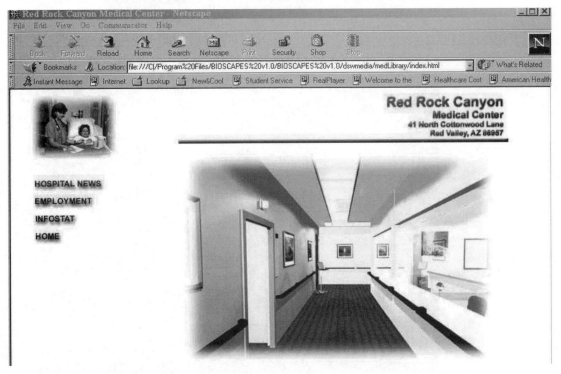

To return to the **Nurses' Station (Room 312)**, exit from the browser. This computer simulates being in a Web environment, so you have to exit from the Intranet by exiting from the browser. Click on **File**, then on **Exit** or **Close** (depending on your browser).

4. Bulletin Board

The bulletin board in the Nurses' Station (Room 312) has important information for students. Click on the board and you can read where reports are being given for patients and where the health team meetings are being held. Lessons in your workbook will direct you to these meetings and reports. Click on **Return** to exit this close-up view of the board.

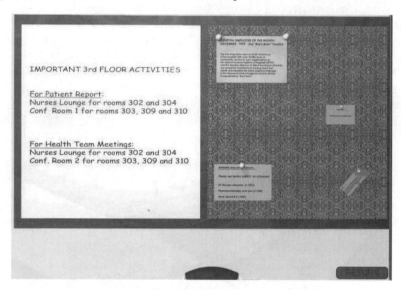

■ VISITING A PATIENT

First, go the Supervisor's Office and sign in to work with Andrea Wang for Tuesday at 0700. Now go to her room. *(Note: The quickest way to get to a patient's room is by double-clicking the room number on the animated map. You can also choose to move through the hallway until you reach the patient's door; then click on the doorknob.)* Once you are inside the room, you will see a still frame of your patient. Below this frame, you will find four icons:

- Vital Signs
- Health History
- Physical
- Medications

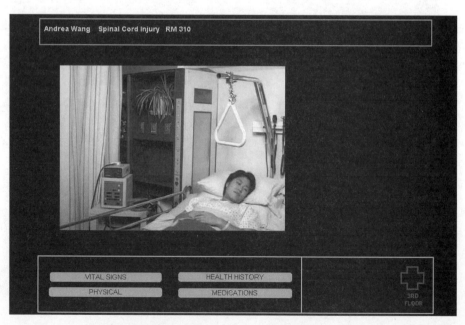

Each of these icons provides the opportunity to assess the patient or the patient's medications. When you click on an icon, you will follow a nurse through the process of collecting assessment data. The nurse will not speak to you but will rely on you to collect the data obtained during patient assessment, to record patient data in the EPR, and sometimes to make decisions after a nurse-patient interaction.

◆   **Vital Signs**

Click on **Vital Signs**; six new icons appear. Each of these new icons allows you to collect data for a particular vital sign. *(Note: You can also see two icons in the right corner. **Continue Working with Patient** takes you back to the main menu for this patient. Clicking on **3rd Floor** will take you back into the hallway.)* Click on the **Temperature** icon. You will see the nurse take the patient's temperature with a tympanic thermometer. At the end of the measurement, the temperature is shown in the animation of the thermometer to the right of the video screen. These types of interactions allow you to collect data during patient visits.

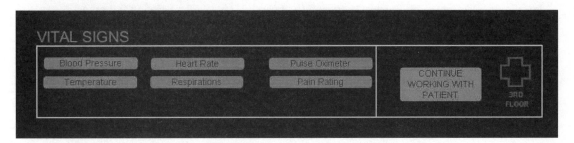

◆   **Physical Examination**

Click **Continue Working with Patient** to return to the main patient menu. Now click the **Physical** icon. Note the different areas of physical examination you can conduct. Try one.

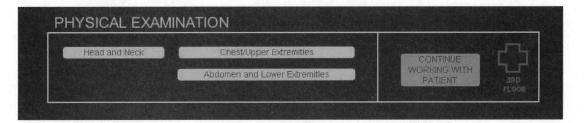

◆   **Health History**

Next, click **Continue Working with Patient** and select the **Health History** icon. In this interactive learning arena, you can ask the patient about her health history. Questions are organized into 12 categories, each of which is accessed by an icon below the video screen. Click on **Culture**, and three new icons appear in the frame to the right of the video. Click on the **Preferred Language** icon, and you will discover the language this patient prefers to use. For each of the 12 question areas, there are three topics you can explore. Thus, there are 36 different question areas related to the health history of each patient.

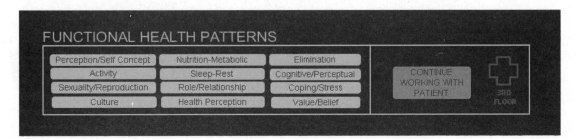

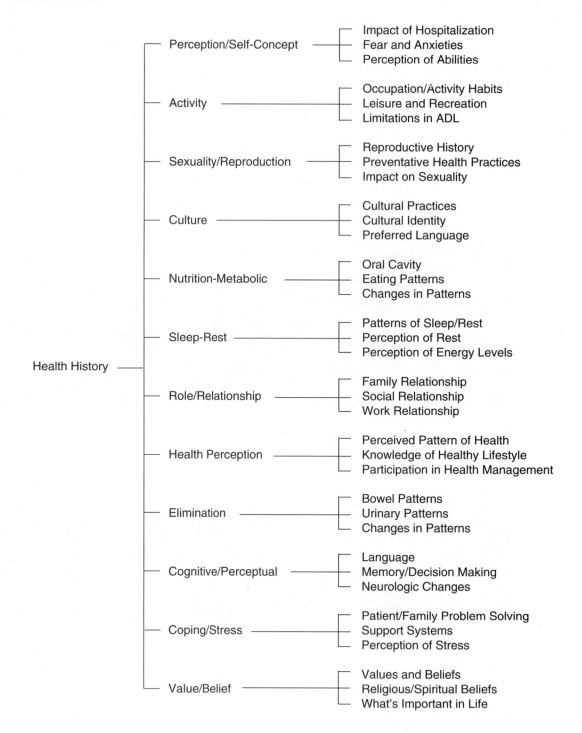

Health History

- Perception/Self-Concept
  - Impact of Hospitalization
  - Fear and Anxieties
  - Perception of Abilities
- Activity
  - Occupation/Activity Habits
  - Leisure and Recreation
  - Limitations in ADL
- Sexuality/Reproduction
  - Reproductive History
  - Preventative Health Practices
  - Impact on Sexuality
- Culture
  - Cultural Practices
  - Cultural Identity
  - Preferred Language
- Nutrition-Metabolic
  - Oral Cavity
  - Eating Patterns
  - Changes in Patterns
- Sleep-Rest
  - Patterns of Sleep/Rest
  - Perception of Rest
  - Perception of Energy Levels
- Role/Relationship
  - Family Relationship
  - Social Relationship
  - Work Relationship
- Health Perception
  - Perceived Pattern of Health
  - Knowledge of Healthy Lifestyle
  - Participation in Health Management
- Elimination
  - Bowel Patterns
  - Urinary Patterns
  - Changes in Patterns
- Cognitive/Perceptual
  - Language
  - Memory/Decision Making
  - Neurologic Changes
- Coping/Stress
  - Patient/Family Problem Solving
  - Support Systems
  - Perception of Stress
- Value/Belief
  - Values and Beliefs
  - Religious/Spiritual Beliefs
  - What's Important in Life

◆   **Medications**

Click **Continue Working with Patient**, and then click the **Medications** icon. Notice that you have three options within this learning environment: Review Medications, Administer, and Hold Medications. Don't click on these now, because you will need to look at this patient's records before you decide whether or not to give medications.

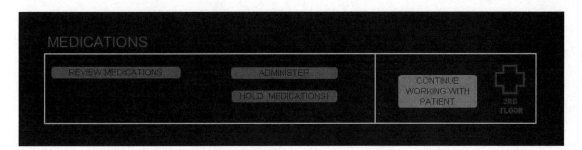

■ HOW TO QUIT OR CHANGE PATIENTS

How to Quit: If necessary, click either the **3rd Floor** icon or the **Nurses' Station** icon (depending on which screen you are currently using) to return to the medical-surgical floor. Then click on the **Quit** icon in the lower right corner of your screen.

How to Change Patients or Shifts: Go to the Supervisor's Office and double-click on the sign-in computer. Click the **Reset** icon. When the next screen appears, select a new patient or a different shift with the same patient.

A DETAILED TOUR ———————————————————————————————————

If you wish to understand the capabilities of the virtual hospital, take a detailed tour by going through the following section.

■ WORKING WITH A PATIENT

Sign in and select Carmen Gonzales as your patient for Tuesday at 0700 hours.

To become more familiar with the *Virtual Clinical Excursions Patients' Disk,* try the following exercises. These activities are designed to introduce you to all of the different components and learning opportunities available within the software. Each exercise will ask you to collect data on a patient.

■ REPORT

In hospitals, when one nurse's shift ends and another begins, the outgoing nurse who attended a patient will give a verbal and sometimes a written summary of that patient's condition to the incoming nurse who will assume care for the patient. This summary is called a *report* and is an important source of data to provide an overview of a patient.

Your first task is to get the report on Carmen Gonzales. Go to the bulletin board in the Nurses' Station. Double-click on the board and check the location where the attending nurse from the previous shift will give you report on this patient. Remember, Carmen Gonzales is in Room 302, so look for that room number on the bulletin board. You will find that the report is being given in the Nurses' Lounge (Room 306). Click **Return** to leave this close-up view of the bulletin board. *(Note: You can also find out where reports are being given by moving your cursor across the animated map.)* Go to Room 306 by double-clicking on the animated map. Once inside the room, click on **Report** and then on **Gonzales**. Listen to report and make a list of this patient's problems and high-priority concerns. When you are finished, click on the **3rd Floor** icon to return to the Nurses' Station.

Problems/Concerns

■ CHARTS

Find the patient charts in the bookshelf to the right of the bulletin board. Double-click on the bookshelf and find Carmen Gonzales' chart (the one labeled **302**). Click on her chart and read the section called Physical & History, including the Emergency Department Record. Determine from this information why Carmen Gonzales has been admitted to the hospital. In the space below, write a brief summary of why this patient was admitted.

■ MEDICATIONS

Open the Medication Administration Record (MAR) by clicking on the blue notebook on the counter of the Nurses' Station. Find the list of medications prescribed for Carmen Gonzales, and write down the medications that need to be given during the time period 0730–0930. For each medication, note dosage, route, and time in the chart below.

Time	Medication	Dosage	Route

Close the MAR and go inside Carmen Gonzales' room (302). Click on the **Medications** icon. You will be responsible for administering the medications ordered during the time period 0730–0930.

To become familiar with the medication options, look at the frame below the video screen. There you will find three opportunities:

- Review Medications
- Administer
- Hold Medications

Click on **Review Medications**. This brings up a frame to the right of the video screen with a list of the medications ordered for the period 0730–0930 hours. Decide whether these medications match what appears within the **Medication Administration Record (MAR)** for this time period. If they do match, you can click the **Administer** icon. If they do not match, you should select **Hold Medications**. When you are finished, click **Continue Working With Patient** to return to the patient care menu.

■ VITAL SIGNS

Vital signs are often considered the traditional signs of life and include body temperature, heart rate, respiratory rate, blood pressure, oxygen saturation of the blood, and the patient's experience of pain.

Inside Carmen Gonzales' room, click on the **Vital Signs** icon. This icon activates a pathway that allows you to measure the patient's vital signs. When you enter this pathway, you will see a short video in which the nurse informs the patient what is about to happen. Six vital signs options appear at the bottom of the screen. Each icon activates a video clip in which the respective vital sign is measured. Relevant vital signs data become available in these videos. For example, click on **Heart Rate**, and a video clip and animation of a radial pulse appear. You can measure the heart rate by counting the animated pulses during a prescribed time.

Try each of the different vital signs options to see what kinds of data are obtained. The vital signs data change over time to reflect the temporal changes you would find in a patient similar to Carmen Gonzales. You will see this most clearly if you "leave" the Tuesday time period you are currently within and "come back" on Thursday. However, you will also find changes throughout any given day (for example, differences between the 0700–1100 and 1100–1500 shifts).

Collect vital signs data for Carmen Gonzales and enter them into the following table. Note the time at which you collected these data.

Vital Signs	Findings/Time
Blood Pressure	
O_2 Saturation	
Heart Rate	
Respiratory Rate	
Temperature	
Pain Rating	

After you are done, click on the **3rd Floor** icon in the lower right portion of your screen. This will take you back into the hallway. Move along the hallway (or use the animated map in the upper right corner of your screen) to return to the Nurses' Station. Enter the station, and click on the computer that accesses the Electronic Patient Record (EPR). First you will see the Electronic Patient Record System entry screen. Type in **rn2b** for the password (remember, do *not* press the Return/Enter key). Then click **Access Records**, and you will see a new screen with patients listed. Click on **Carmen Gonzales** and then on **Access EPR**. Now you are in the EPR system. Click on **Vital Signs**, which will open the screen with vital signs data. Use the blue and orange arrows in the lower right-hand corner of the data table to move around within the database. Look at the data collected earlier for each of the vital signs you measured. Use these data to establish a baseline for each of the vital signs.

a. Are any of the data you collected significantly different from the baselines for those vital signs?	Circle One: Yes No
b. If "Yes," which data are different?	

PHYSICAL ASSESSMENT

After examining the EPR for vital signs, click the **Assessment** icon and review Carmen Gonzales' data in this area. Once you have reviewed the data and noted any areas of concern to you, close the EPR, enter Carmen Gonzales' room, and click on the **Physical** icon. This will activate the following three options for conducting a physical assessment of the patient:

- Head and Neck
- Chest/Upper Extremities
- Abdomen and Lower Extremities

Click on the **Head and Neck** icon. You will see the nurse conduct an assessment of the head and neck. At the end of the video, a series of icons appear in a frame to the right of the video screen. These icons list the different areas of the head and neck that were examined and the data obtained during the examination. The icons allow you to replay that section of the video in which the particular area was examined.

For example, if you click on **Oculomotor** (the finding is "Oculomotor function intact"), you will see a replay of the assessment of oculomotor function. Each of the icons activates only that portion of the head and neck assessment focused on the particular area described by the icon. The intention is to help you correlate each part of a physical assessment with the data obtained from that assessment—and to give you the opportunity to have the whole assessment of a region conducted beginning to end so that you can learn the process as well as its component parts. Click **Continue Working with Patient** and explore the Chest/Upper Extremities and the Abdomen and Lower Extremities options. For each area, browse through the icons that provide data on a particular area of the assessment. *(Note: The data for certain attributes found during physical assessments change for some patients as you follow them through the virtual week.)*

Focus on the examination of the abdomen and lower extremities by clicking on the option. Pay close attention to the leg wound. In the following table, record the data collected by the nurse during the examination.

Area of Examination	Findings
Abdomen	
Legs	

After you have completed the physical examination of the abdomen and lower extremities, click **Continue Working with Patient** to return to the patient care menu. From there, click on the **3rd Floor** icon and return to the Nurses' Station. Enter the data you collected in Carmen Gonzales' EPR. Compare the data that were already in the record with the data you just collected.

a. Are any of the data you collected significantly different from the baselines for those vital signs?	Circle One: Yes No
b. If "Yes," which data are different?	

■ HEALTH HISTORY

Conduct part of a health history of Carmen Gonzales. Return to her room and click on the **Health History** icon. Twelve health history areas become visible as icons below the video screen. For example, you can see Perception/Self-Concept, Activity, Sexuality/Reproduction, and so on. Note that this patient speaks Spanish and that the nurse has brought in a translator. All of the health history conversations with Carmen Gonzales are completed through translation. Clicking on any of the 12 health history icons reveals three question areas for that category. For example, if you click **Perception/Self-Concept**, a box appears to the right of the video screen with three question areas:

- Impact of Hospitalization
- Fear and Anxieties
- Perception of Abilities

Each of these three areas can be activated by clicking on their respective icons. When an icon is clicked, you will see a video in which your preceptor asks a question in the respective area and the patient answers through the translator.

Since there are 12 health history areas, with three areas of questioning for each, you have access to a total of 36 video clips that provide an opportunity to learn quite a bit about Carmen Gonzales. The questions and responses were chosen for reasons. In fact, conducting an actual health history would not unfold in such discrete and isolated moments; in the real world you would need to follow up some responses with additional questions. Other lessons in this workbook will encourage you to look at each of the health history areas and decide what additional questions need to be asked.

Unlike the vital signs and physical examination findings, the health history data do not change. The developers of *Virtual Clinical Excursions* realized that the number of videos (and the space required for storage) would become too large for the type of educational package we envisioned. We therefore decided to produce only one set of health history data-collecting opportunities. In truth, the health history would probably not change much over a week. Lessons in your workbook may have you collect health history data on the first day of care, or some of the health history queries may be assigned for Tuesday and the others for Thursday.

We recommend that you explore the health history of Carmen Gonzales by choosing some of the 12 categories and asking one or two of the three questions available for each area. When you are done exploring the health history options, leave the patient's room and go to one of the computers that allow you to access the EPR. Browse through the different data fields to see where you would enter data from the health history questions.

Remember: When you are ready to stop working with your *Virtual Clinical Excursions Patients' Disk*, click on the **Quit** icon found in the lower right-hand corner of any of the 3rd floor screens.

■ COLLECTING AND EVALUATING DATA

Each of the patient care activities generates a great deal of assessment data. Remember that after you collect data, you can go to the Nurses' Station or the mobile computer outside Room 302 and enter the data into the EPR. You also can review the data in the EPR, as well as review a patient's chart and MAR. You will get plenty of practice collecting and then evaluating data in the context of the patient's course during previous shifts.

Now, here's an important question for you:

> Did the previous sequence of exercises provide the most efficient way to assess Carmen Gonzales?

For example, you went to the patient's room to get vital signs, then back to the EPR to enter data and your finding with extant data. Then, you went back to the patient's room to do a physical examination, and again back to the EPR to enter and review data. If this back-and-forth process of data collection and recording seemed inefficient, remember the following:

- You want to plan all of your nursing activities to maximize efficiency while at the same time optimizing quality of patient care.
- You collect a tremendous amount of data when you work with a patient. Very few people can accurately remember all these data for more than a few minutes. Develop efficient assessment skills, and enter assessment data as soon as possible after collecting them.
- Assessment data are only the starting point for the nursing process.

Make a clear distinction between these first exercises and how you actually provide nursing care. These initial exercises were designed to involve you actively in the use of different software components. This workbook focuses on sensible practices for implementing the nursing process in ways that ensure the highest quality care of patients.

Most importantly, remember that a human being changes through time—and that these changes include both the physical and psychosocial facets of a person as a living organism. Think about this for a moment. Some patients may change physically in a very short time (a patient with emerging myocardial infarction) or more slowly (a patient with chronic illness). Patients' overall physical and psychosocial conditions may improve or deteriorate. They may have effective coping skills and familial support or feel they are alone and full of despair. In fact, each individual is a complex mix of physical and psychosocial elements, and at least some of these elements usually change through time.

Thus it is crucial *not* to think of the nursing process as a simple one-time, five-step procedure:

- Assessment
- Nursing Diagnosis
- Planning
- Implementation
- Evaluation

Rather, it is a creative and systematic approach to delivering nursing care. Furthermore, because all living organisms are constantly changing, we must apply the nursing process over and over. Each time we follow the nursing process for an individual patient, we refine our understanding of that patient's physical and psychosocial conditions based on collection and analyses of many different types of data. *Virtual Clinical Excursions* will help you develop both the creativity and the systematic approach needed to become a nurse who can deliver the highest quality care to all patients.

The following icons are used throughout the workbook to help you quickly identify particular activities and assignments:

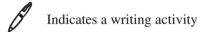 Indicates a reading assignment—tells you which textbook chapter(s) you should read before starting each lesson

Indicates a writing activity

Marks the beginning of an interactive CD-ROM activity—signals you to open or return to your *Virtual Clinical Excursions Patients' Disk*

Indicates additional CD-ROM instructions

Indicates questions and activities that require you to consult your textbook

LESSON 1

Critical Thinking and Nursing Judgment

👓 **Reading Assignment:** Critical Thinking and Nursing Judgment (Chapter 13)
Nursing Assessment (Chapter 14)

Patients: Carmen Gonzales, Room 302
Andrea Wang, Room 310

Objectives

- Identify how the nurse applies critical thinking to the assessment of a patient.
- Apply diagnostic reasoning in the case studies.
- Identify examples of critical thinking attitudes applied in the assessment of patients' health histories in the case studies.
- Discuss the intellectual standards used in the nurse's line of questioning during assessment of patients' health histories.
- Apply critical thinking to the nursing process in the case studies.

When patients seek health care, they depend on nurses to be able to think critically and to perform in a compassionate and professional manner. Critical thinking is so essential to your ability to recognize a patient's needs and to identify the best way to provide therapeutic intervention. Throughout any encounter with a patient, you must always use the skills of critical thinking: recalling past experiences that can help in the care of your current patient, reflecting on the knowledge that applies to a given patient's clinical condition, and anticipating and then applying the intellectual standards and attitudes needed to perform a complete patient assessment. As a critical thinker, you will always ask, "Do I know enough about this patient?" "What do the patient's behaviors mean?" "Are there other sources of information I need to go to?" "Are my conclusions accurate, and if not, how do I gather further information?" The exercises within this lesson will help you learn more about critical thinking and understand how basic this skill is to making sound nursing judgments for your patients.

Exercise 1 – Carmen Gonzales, Thursday 1100

 Let's begin in Room 301, the Supervisor's Office. First, click on the sign-in computer on the supervisor's desk. Enter your name and student ID when prompted; then click **Continue**. Select Carmen Gonzales as your patient for the Thursday 1100 shift. Exit the Supervisor's Office and turn to your left. Go down the hall to the Nurses' Station and check on the bulletin board for the location of the nursing report on Carmen Gonzales (the nurse's lounge, Room 306). Go to Room 306 and listen to the report. *(Note: You can also navigate by using the animated map in the upper right corner of your screen.)*

1. Complete the following form as you take notes from the report on Carmen Gonzales.

   Diagnosis(es):

   Vital Signs: BP _____   RR ____   HR ____   Temp ____ O_2 Sat ____

   Recent Medications:

   Physical Findings:

   Lab Results:

2. Match each of the following assessment data with the corresponding intellectual standard, to describe how the nurse's report on Carmen Gonzales' lungs could be more thorough.

Standard	Assessment Data
_____ Specific	a. Additional description if there is a productive cough
_____ Accurate	b. Description of portion of lung involved
_____ Broad	c. Description of extent of congestion through reporting the type of adventitious lung sounds

3. Which of the following intellectual standards is met in the nurse's report of vital signs?
   a. Precise
   b. Consistent
   c. Relevant
   d. Logical

➡ Now exit Room 306 and go to one of the computers that allow you to access the Electronic Patient Record (EPR): either the desktop computer under the bookshelf in the Nurses' Station or the mobile computer next to Room 302. Open Carmen Gonzales' EPR; then click on **Admissions** to review her Admissions Profile.

4. Now that you have read the Admissions Profile, you know that Carmen Gonzales has diabetes. The serious gangrenous infection of her foot is a result of poor control of her disease. She states in the record that she does not understand why her foot is infected. The entry in the chart recommending diabetes education is an example of:

   a. nursing diagnosis.

   b. reflection.

   c. clinical decision making.

   d. intuition.

5. An important part of critical thinking is to draw upon your knowledge base when assessing patient needs. As you review the Admissions Profile for Carmen Gonzales, what areas of knowledge do you believe are important to apply in order to more thoroughly assess whether diabetes education is appropriate?

6. Carmen Gonzales' Admissions Profile notes that the patient has pain in the left leg, the site of infection. For each of the following intellectual standards, identify the types of assessment questions you might ask to get a better understanding of this patient's pain.

   a. Clear:

   b. Relevant:

   c. Precise:

   d. Consistent:

→ Exit the EPR and go to Room 302 to visit Carmen Gonzales. Begin by reviewing her health history. Once you have selected **Health History**, click on **Perception/Self-Concept**. Then click on each of the three question areas (one at a time) to observe the nurse's assessment.

7. During the assessment of the Perception/Self-Concept category, how might the nurse have demonstrated perseverance when assessing Carmen Gonzales' fears?

→ Click on **Sexuality/Reproduction** and observe this assessment by selecting the various question areas.

8. Risk taking generally comes with experience but shows your willingness to take an extra step even if the results can be undesirable. How did the nurse use risk taking when assessing Carmen Gonzales' sexuality?

➤ Next, conduct a focused review on the following categories and question areas: Perception/Self-Concept—Fears and Anxieties; Activity—Limitations in ADL; Coping/Stress—Perception of Stress; and Value/Belief—What's Important in Life.

9. Based on the information you have just reviewed, describe what you think might be Carmen Gonzales' psychosocial problem or concern.

➤ Now review these health history areas: Nutrition-Metabolic—Eating Patterns; Health Perception—Knowledge of Healthy Lifestyle and Participation in Health Management.

10. It is important to interpret data from the health history along with what you learned earlier in the Admissions Profile about Carmen Gonzales' medical history and complications with diabetes. She seems to be a candidate for diabetes education, but you need to assess more. This requires critical thinking—using knowledge, experience, attitudes and standards. Complete the following critical thinking diagram for assessment by writing the letter of each critical thinking factor under its corresponding category.

KNOWLEDGE

(1) _____

(2) _____

(3) _____

EXPERIENCE	**ASSESSMENT OF DIABETES EDUCATION**	**STANDARDS**
(4) _____		(5) _____
		(6) _____

ATTITUDES

(7) _____

(8) _____

Critical Thinking Factors

    a. Find a way to better confirm what Carmen Gonzales eats daily (e.g., ask husband to keep a food diary).

    b. Reflect on the time you have spent observing a dietitian present a nutrition class to patients with diabetes.

    c. Review standards for patient education from the American Diabetes Association.

    d. Components of a diabetic diet.

    e. Ask a diabetes nurse specialist to give you information about what to assess regarding Carmen Gonzales' dietary habits.

    f. Influence of health beliefs on motivation to learn.

    g. Spend more time asking Carmen Gonzales to describe what she knows about diabetes.

    h. Cultural influence on learning health promotion practices.

11. An important part of assessment is the nurse's skill in the use of interview techniques. Review the nurse's assessment of Carmen Gonzales' nutrition; then match each of the following nurse's questions with the corresponding interview technique. (More than one question may apply to each technique.)

Interview Technique	Nurse's Question
_____ Open-ended question	a. "Do you still have teeth?"
_____ Closed-ended question	b. "Tell me what you eat for breakfast."
	c. "What are your favorite foods?"

12. An important aspect of critical thinking is interpretation of data. Review findings from the assessment of Carmen Gonzales' perception/self-concept and health perception. What interpretations can you make?

13. What further information would you want to assess?

→ Exit the patient's room and go to the Nurses' Station. Open Carmen Gonzales' chart and click on **Nurses' Notes**. Read the notes for Sunday at 2100.

14. Does the entry listed under Subjective Data meet the criteria for the definition of *subjective data*? Explain.

Exercise 2 – Andrea Wang, Tuesday 1100

 Return to the Supervisor's Office to sign in for a new patient. After clicking on the desktop computer, you will need to click on the **Reset** icon. Then select Andrea Wang for Tuesday at 1100. Now go to the Nurses' Station and review her EPR, specifically the Admissions Profile. Exit the EPR and go inside Andrea Wang's room. Click on **Health History**; then observe the nurse's assessment of each of the 12 health history categories.

1. From the assessment of the 12 categories covering Andrea Wang's health history, match each of the following questions or statements with the corresponding communication strategy.

Communication Strategy	**Nurse's Question or Statement**
_____ Closed-ended question	a. "Tell me how you are doing today."
_____ Offering information	b. "How does that make you feel?"
_____ Focused question	c. "You know, Andrea, an accident like this can cause problems and changes in your bowel and bladder function. We can talk about that if you like."
_____ Open-ended question	
	d. "Do you feel rested?"

2. Part of critical thinking and assessment is the collection of data and the organization of data into meaningful clusters. As you listen to Andrea Wang's health history interview, you should hear cues that start to show a pattern. Match each of the following cues with the corresponding pattern. (More than one cue may be matched with a pattern.)

Pattern	**Cue**
_____ Anger	a. "Well, you know, I've led an active life. I can't believe this is happening."
_____ Grief over loss	b. "Deep down I feel exhausted and helpless."
_____ Hopelessness	c. "I've been in good health—hardly ever got sick, but now I feel lost."
	d. "Well, not much. We're hoping the paralysis isn't permanent."
	e. "I don't know what's going to happen to them—and me."
	f. "I just want to be able to walk around."
	g. "Not unless you'll tell me I'll stop being incontinent in a few days."

3. Grief over loss of body function is common with an acute spinal cord injury. You have begun to recognize cues in the data Andrea Wang has shared. However, you need to learn more. Complete the following critical thinking diagram for assessment of grief by writing the letter of each critical thinking factor under its corresponding category.

KNOWLEDGE

(1) _____

(2) _____

(3) _____

EXPERIENCE	ASSESSMENT OF GRIEF	STANDARDS
(4) _____		(6) _____
(5) _____		(7) _____

ATTITUDES

(8) _____

(9) _____

Critical Thinking Factors

    a. Ask Andrea Wang if you can interview her boyfriend Eric and discuss how he feels about her injury.

    b. Review information about the stages of grief.

    c. Explore more into Andrea Wang's feelings about her accident.

    d. Determine the physiologic effects of a spinal cord transection.

    e. Recommend a family conference to learn about mother's and father's attitudes and feelings about the care their daughter will need at home.

    f. Consider a time when you have had a personal loss and how it made you feel.

    g. Clarify how Andrea Wang normally slept when at home.

    h. Review your journal notes taken when you cared for a patient who had lost function in the right arm.

    i. Review the theory of developmental needs of young adults.

4. One concern Andrea Wang alludes to in her assessment is her difficulty imagining that she will be in a wheelchair. Part of a nurse's assessment is a review of a patient's environmental history. What might be useful to collect in Andrea Wang's case?

2

Applying the Nursing Process

∽∞ **Reading Assignment:** Nursing Assessment (Chapter 14)
Nursing Diagnosis (Chapter 15)
Planning for Nursing Care (Chapter 16)
Implementing Nursing Care (Chapter 17)
Evaluation (Chapter 18)

Patients: David Ruskin, Room 303
Andrea Wang, Room 310

Objectives

- Assess the health care needs of patients in the case studies.
- Form data clusters from information interpreted in a nursing assessment.
- Demonstrate how physical assessment data confirms information from the health history.
- Develop nursing diagnoses from data presented in the case studies.
- Apply critical thinking to the nursing diagnostic process.
- Identify priorities of nursing care for patients in the case studies.
- Develop outcome statements.
- Develop a nursing plan of care.
- Identify types of nursing interventions.
- Select evaluation methods appropriate to a patient's plan of care.
- Evaluate a plan of care

As a nurse, you will routinely apply the nursing process as you diagnose and treat your patients' responses to health and illness. Whether you care for a patient who suffers a life-threatening illness or you are counseling a mother with a new baby, the nursing process becomes your "set of tools" for ensuring that you know your patients' needs, selecting the right nursing therapies, administering your care, and evaluating its effectiveness. At first you will find yourself thinking very logically and systematically as you apply the nursing process in the care of patients. Each step of the process is a methodical and orderly approach to critical thinking. Eventually, as you acquire more experience the nursing process becomes an automatic way of thinking critically and acting as a competent professional.

Exercise 1 – David Ruskin, Tuesday 1100

 Go to the Supervisor's Office and sign in to work with David Ruskin on Tuesday at 1100. Proceed to the bulletin board in the Nurses' Station to find out where his change-of-shift report is being given (Room 307). Go to Room 307 and listen to the report. *(Note: You can also find out where report is being given by moving your cursor across the animated map.)*

1. Complete the following form as you listen to report on David Ruskin.

Patient's Name:

Diagnosis:

Vital Signs: BP _____ RR ____ HR ____ Temp ____ O$_2$ Sat ____

Patient Data (Signs and Symptoms):

Mental Status:

---

2. As you review the patient data reported for David Ruskin, identify whether each of the following findings is an example of subjective data (mark with an **S**) or objective data (mark with an **O**).

_____ Pain in left arm and side

_____ States hurts some to breathe

_____ Has lot of aches and pains

_____ Lungs clear

_____ Alert and oriented to person and place

3. Following report, you should organize the data you received about David Ruskin so that you will know how to continue your assessment when you visit him in his room. Classify the data from report by writing each piece of data next to the appropriate heading below.

Circulation:

Respiration:

Comfort:

Skin:

4. From the initial data available on David Ruskin, you will begin to think of questions to ask him to clarify, broaden, and confirm what you know. Given the following data, identify questions that you might ask to improve your data base.

Data   **Questions to Ask**

Respiration
   Lungs clear
   Breathing regular
   Hurts some to breathe

Comfort
   Pain in left arm and side
   States he has a lot of aches and pains
   Hurts some to breathe

Skin
   IV in left hand
   Abrasions present, no infection

5. As you review David Ruskin's assessment data by system classification, identify three areas that suggest a pattern of potential problems.

   a.

   b.

   c.

→ Now exit the report room, return to the Nurses' Station, and access David Ruskin's EPR. To gather additional assessment data, click on **Vital Signs**, **Admissions**, and **Assessment** and review each of these sections.

6. The information you learned from the EPR adds to your data base. Record this additional information as data clusters next to the three potential problem areas identified in question 5 (from change-of-shift report).

Data Clusters

Pain

Difficulty Breathing

Potential Infection

→ Now you are ready to visit David Ruskin. Go to his room (303) and observe the nurse as she assesses his vital signs (specifically pain assessment) and performs his physical examination.

7. To determine a basis for comparing David Ruskin's pain over time, the nurse uses which objective standard?
   a. Asking the patient to locate the pain
   b. Using a pain rating scale
   c. Observing the patient's nonverbal expression of pain
   d. Observing the patient's body movements

8. After reviewing the data on David Ruskin, you began to form clusters of information that reveal problem areas. On the basis of your findings, match each of the following defining characteristics with the corresponding nursing diagnosis. (Each diagnosis will have more than one defining characteristic.)

Defining Characteristic	Nursing Diagnosis
_____ Verbal report of discomfort (I feel sharp pain in the chest when I take a deep breath)	a. Ineffective Breathing Pattern
_____ Depth of breathing (respirations guarded on admission)	b. Pain
_____ Chest hurts when he takes deep breath	
_____ Moans and groans when arm moved	
_____ Pain rating of 7	
_____ Respiratory pattern shallow	

9. As you apply critical thinking to the formation of the nursing diagnosis of Pain, complete the critical thinking diagram below by writing the letter of each critical thinking factor under its corresponding category.

KNOWLEDGE

(1) _____

(2) _____

(3) _____

EXPERIENCE	**NURSING DIAGNOSIS FOR DAVID RUSKIN: PAIN**	**STANDARDS**
(4) _____		(5) _____
		(6) _____

ATTITUDES

(7) _____

(8) _____

Critical Thinking Factors

    a. Pain assessment using a visual analog scale will precisely measure pain intensity.
    b. Show discipline in taking time to thoroughly assess all factors that affect the patient's pain.
    c. The pathology of rib and cartilage injury explains the nature of David Ruskin's chest pain.
    d. Caring for patients with orthopedic injuries will assist you in assessing David Ruskin's pain.
    e. The natural healing process following repair of a fractured humerus will allow you to anticipate the type of discomfort David Ruskin will experience.
    f. Because David Ruskin is very active, your assessment should include how pain affects the activities he most enjoys.
    g. As you perform an assessment, show the patient how to correctly move and reposition so as to cause the least discomfort.
    h. Apply what you know about the character of pain to ensure your assessment is thorough.

10. A nursing diagnostic statement contains a two-part diagnostic statement. In the case of David Ruskin, he is experiencing pain related to:
    a. open reduction and fixation of humerus.
    b. limited movement of arm.
    c. surgical trauma to muscles and tissues in right arm and physical trauma to chest.
    d. recovery from bike injury.

11. The nurse writes the following nursing diagnosis: Pain related to open reduction and fixation of humerus. What type of diagnostic error does this diagnosis contain?
    a. Identifies a clinical sign
    b. Identifies the nurse's problem
    c. Identifies a medical diagnosis
    d. Identifies a nursing intervention

12. Explain the difference between an actual health problem such as David Ruskin's pain and an at-risk health problem.

13. Given the risk factors of broken skin, traumatized tissue, and an invasive procedure (IV insertion), what nursing diagnosis would apply to David Ruskin's situation?

14. From a review of David Ruskin's clinical data, you have identified three nursing diagnoses: Risk for infection; Ineffective breathing pattern; and Pain. Order these three diagnoses by priority and provide a rationale for your decision.

15. For the nursing diagnosis of pain, develop one goal of care for David Ruskin, making sure it is patient-centered, singular, and time-limited.

16. Expected outcomes are the specific, step-by-step objectives that lead to attainment of the goal of care. Which of the following is a properly written expected outcome relating to the goal of pain relief for David Ruskin?
    a. Patient will have better ability to breathe deeply.
    b. Patient will move about more freely in bed.
    c. Patient will use fewer analgesics over the next 24 hours.
    d. Patient will report pain acuity ≤4 on a scale of 0 to 10.

17. Based on what you know about David Ruskin, write a goal and two outcomes of care for the following nursing diagnosis: Ineffective breathing pattern related to chest pain.

    Goal:

    Outcomes:

→ Now leave the patient's room and go to the Nurses' Station. Open David Ruskin's chart and read the physician's orders and the nurses' notes.

18. Identify from the chart two physician-initiated interventions for David Ruskin's pain.

19. The nurses' notes do not reveal a nursing plan of care for David Ruskin's chest or arm pain. Indicate whether each of the following interventions would be nurse-initiated (mark with an **N**) or physician-initiated (mark with a **P**).

_____   Change analgesic route from intravenous to oral.

_____   Splint right chest during coughing.

_____   Have patient perform relaxation exercises when analgesic is given.

_____   Offer analgesic 30 minutes before ambulation or ADL.

_____   Order chest x-ray if pain increases.

➡ Return to the Supervisor's Office and select David Ruskin as your patient for the Thursday 0700 shift. Next, go to one of the computers from which you can access the EPR. Open David Ruskin's EPR and review his assessment data for Wednesday evening through Thursday morning.

20. It is important to determine whether interventions are effective in resolving a patient's health problem. Identify three evaluation measures you could use to determine David Ruskin's response to pain management therapy.

21. Based on the information in David Ruskin's EPR, compare his assessment and vital signs data for Wednesday at 2400 with data for Tuesday at 1600. Answer each of the following questions by circling the correct choice.

a. Has his chest expansion improved?   Yes   No   Unchanged

b. Has the intensity of pain been reduced?   Yes   No   Unchanged

c. Is movement pain-free?   Yes   No

d. Is the respiratory pattern normal?   Yes   No

22. Based on your evaluation findings, what should be your next course of action?
a. Continue current plan of care.
b. Continue therapies that are effective and consider adding interventions to reduce pain during positioning and movement.
c. Continue therapies that are effective and consider adding interventions to reduce pain during coughing.
d. Discontinue current plan of care.

Exercise 2 –Andrea Wang, Tuesday 1100

Go to the Supervisor's Office and sign in to work with Andrea Wang on Tuesday at 1100. Next, find out where the nurse from the previous shift is giving report on this patient (Room 307). Go to that location and listen to report.

1. Based on the information shared during report, identify three areas of need that you would like to assess more thoroughly when you meet Andrea Wang.

   a.

   b.

   c.

2. To assess Andrea Wang in a thorough manner and to learn as much as you can about her health status, apply the critical thinking model. Complete the diagram below by writing the letter of each critical thinking factor under its corresponding category.

KNOWLEDGE

(1) _____

(2) _____

EXPERIENCE

(3) _____

**ASSESSMENT OF
ANDREA WANG**

STANDARDS

(4) _____

(5) _____

ATTITUDES

(6) _____

(7) _____

Critical Thinking Factors
   a. Consider use of a family conference to gain more information about the patient.
   b. Effect of spinal cord transection on motor and sensory function.
   c. Respect the patient's right to know about family conference and to decide whether it is acceptable.
   d. Communication skills needed to convey caring and interest in Andrea Wang's condition.
   e. Effect of experiencing a personal loss.
   f. Display an understanding of Andrea Wang's condition and a willingness to work with her in identifying the best treatment plan.
   g. Conduct a complete assessment of Andrea Wang's acceptance of her injury.

→ Now go inside Room 310 to visit Andrea Wang. Review the entire health history, paying attention not only to what the patient says but also to the way in which she communicates with the nurse.

3. As you review the health history, use the space below to collect notes on the three areas of need you identified for Andrea Wang in question 1.

   Sleep:

   Support from family/friends:

   Coping with stress of injury:

4. Given the information you have gathered about Andrea Wang, identify three nursing diagnoses that apply. Defend your decision by listing two or three defining characteristics for each diagnosis.

   Diagnosis   **Defining Characteristics**

5. Are there additional problem areas you began to identify while listening to Andrea Wang's health history? If so, which of the following nursing diagnoses best describe her situation?
   a. Hopelessness; Altered nutrition: less than body requirements; Body image disturbance
   b. Pain; Bowel incontinence; Risk for impaired skin integrity
   c. Self-esteem disturbance; Hopelessness; Loneliness
   d. Bowel incontinence; Risk for impaired skin integrity; Anxiety

6. For the nursing diagnosis of Impaired skin integrity, identify a goal of care and two expected outcomes for Andrea Wang. *(Study Tip: See Chapter 47 in your textbook.)*

Goal

Outcomes

7. For the nursing diagnosis of Ineffective individual coping, list two approaches you might use to evaluate Andrea Wang's response to nursing care.

LESSON 3

Caring in the Practice Setting

 Reading Assignment: Nursing Healing and Caring (Chapter 6)

Patients: Andrea Wang, Room 310
Ira Bradley, Room 309

Objectives

- Identify nursing approaches used in the case studies that display the five caring processes defined by Swanson.
- Describe how to convey comforting during a physical examination.
- Identify strategies to be able to "know" a patient.
- Describe how the nurse might include family to enhance caring in the case studies.

You have already learned that caring is more than a simple feeling of benevolence towards another individual. Caring is the essence of what we, as nurses, do for our patients. Caring means being connected with, doing for, and being with an individual during a time of vulnerability and infirmity. As you go through the following exercises, you will gain a better sense of how nurses demonstrate caring in their practice. In addition, you will see opportunities where caring behaviors might be enhanced for given patients.

Exercise 1 – Andrea Wang, Tuesday 1100

Begin by going to the Supervisor's Office and signing in to work with Andrea Wang on Tuesday at 1100. Then go to the Nurses' Station and find her chart. Checking a patient's medical history is often one of the first things a nurse does in preparing to know and care for a patient. To accomplish this, open Andrea Wang's chart and review the nurses' notes and the Physical & History. (Remember to scroll down to read all pages.) Now that you know a little bit about this patient, proceed to her room (310) and go inside.

1. First observe Andrea Wang as she lies in bed. What do you notice that conveys a sense of comforting?

2. Click on **Vital Signs** and observe the nurse's approach prior to the measurement of Andrea Wang's vital signs. Which of the following behaviors communicate a sense of presence to the patient? (Place an **X** next to all correct answers.)

_____ Calling the patient by her name

_____ Using a calm tone of voice

_____ Providing a gentle touch

_____ Acquiring the patient's consent

_____ Standing close to the patient's side

_____ Maintaining eye contact with the patient

➡ When you have finished measuring vital signs, click on **Continue Working with Patient**, then click on **Physical**. Begin the physical examination with the head and neck. Then move to the chest and upper extremities and finish with the abdomen and lower extremities.

3. As you observe the nurse, watch for behaviors that represent the subdimensions of "doing for" and "enabling," as described in Swanson's theory of caring. Place an **X** next to all of the following subdimensions that apply for each caring process.

Caring Processes   **Subdimensions**

"Doing For"   _____ Comforting

                                  _____ Anticipating

                                  _____ Performing skillfully

                                  _____ Protecting

                                  _____ Preserving dignity

"Enabling"   _____ Informing/explaining

                                  _____ Supporting/allowing

                                  _____ Focusing

                                  _____ Generating alternatives

                                  _____ Validating/giving feedback

4. If you were the nurse caring for Andrea Wang, what might you have done differently during the examination that would better demonstrate "enabling"?

→ Continue working with the patient. This time, click on the **Health History** icon and observe the nurse's assessment of Andrea Wang by selecting the three question areas under the categories of Perception/Self-Concept and Value/Belief.

5. Now that you have observed the health history, critique the nurse's success in getting to "know" Andrea Wang:

   a. Explain the significance of the nurse's question, "How does that make you feel?"

   b. List three questions you might ask Andrea Wang that would allow you to better learn about her values and beliefs.

Exercise 2 – Ira Bradley, Thursday 1100

 Go to the Supervisor's Office and sign in to work the Thursday 1100 shift with Ira Bradley as your patient. Then go to one of the computers that allow you to access the EPR. Open Ira Bradley's EPR, click on **Admissions**, and review his Admissions Profile carefully. This patient has an advanced case of human immunodeficiency virus (HIV) infection. At the time of admission, he was confused and unable to respond to the questions reliably. The Admissions Profile gives you a summary of how his wife answered the initial admission history questions. Once you have read the Admissions Profile, exit the EPR and go to the Nurses' Station. Open Ira Bradley's chart and review the nurses' notes. As you read the notes, you will find that he has shown some improvement in orientation and his overall appetite. Now close the chart and go into Room 309 to meet Ira Bradley and his wife.

1. Observe the patient's physical examination, comparing the nurse's style with that of the nurse observed in Exercise 1. Describe ways in which Ira Bradley's nurse demonstrated "doing for" during the physical examination.

2. Now observe the complete health history conducted with Ira Bradley and his wife. Identify three ways in which the nurse failed to demonstrate caring towards this family.

3. Swanson's theory of caring describes "maintaining belief." Now that you have listened to Ira Bradley describe his condition, which of the following caring subdimension do you feel will be the most challenging for the nurse to provide?
   a. Believing in/holding esteem
   b. Maintaining a hope-filled attitude
   c. Offering realistic optimism
   d. "Going the distance"

4. Ira Bradley's condition is terminal, and he knows he is dying. In what ways can the nurse provide hope or a degree of realistic optimism?

5. Family care is a part of caring for an individual patient. During the nurse's assessment of Ira Bradley's elimination status, which of the following of Mayer's 10 nurse caring behaviors should the nurse have provided? (Circle all correct answers.)

   a. Being honest

   b. Giving clear explanations

   c. Keeping the family informed

   d. Trying to make patient comfortable

   e. Showing interest in answering questions

   f. Providing necessary emergency care

   g. Assuring the patient that nursing services will be available

   h. Allowing the patient to do things for himself

   i. Teaching the family how to keep the patient physically comfortable

Exercise 3 – Ira Bradley, Thursday 1100 (continued)

 Exit Ira Bradley's room and go to Room 308 to attend the health team meeting. Listen to each team member's report. Then go to the Nurses' Station and open Ira Bradley's chart. Click on **Health Team** and review each member's written report.

1. In the case manager's written report, which dimension of Swanson's caring theory was best addressed in the plan of care?
   a. Knowing
   b. Being with
   c. Doing for
   d. Enabling
   e. Maintaining belief

2. In what way does the clinical nurse specialist's plan support efforts to display hope for Ira Bradley?

Exercise 4 – Andrea Wang and Ira Bradley, Thursday 1100

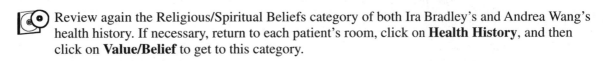 Review again the Religious/Spiritual Beliefs category of both Ira Bradley's and Andrea Wang's health history. If necessary, return to each patient's room, click on **Health History**, and then click on **Value/Belief** to get to this category.

1. What do Andrea Wang and Ira Bradley have in common, thereby making spiritual caring especially important?

 Study Tip: To review possible nursing approaches for spiritual caring, review Chapter 28 in your textbook.

Physical Examination and Vital Signs

Reading Assignment: Vital Signs (Chapter 31
Health Assessment and Physical Examination (Chapter 32))

Patients: Sally Begay, Room 304
Ira Bradley, Room 309

Objectives

- Critique the approaches used in the case studies for conducting a physical examination and measuring vital signs.
- Explain why certain physical examination techniques are used with patients in the case studies.
- Discuss how changes resulting from disease or injury might affect physical examination findings and vital signs.
- Discuss how nursing therapies might change physical examination findings.

The use of skillful techniques in conducting a physical examination and measuring vital signs gives you a valuable set of tools for assessing a patient's condition. Findings from an examination help to determine the patient's needs and the types of nursing therapies most appropriate. After you administer nursing therapies, physical examination and vital sign measurement can help you to evaluate how the patient responds and determine whether the plan of care can continue or should be revised. The exercises in this lesson will give you a clear sense for how physical examination and vital sign measurement become incorporated into a nurse's daily routine and how approaches are individualized based on a patient's history and presenting condition. This lesson also gives you an opportunity to compare examination approaches based upon different patients' presenting symptoms.

Exercise 1 – Sally Begay, Tuesday 1100

Go to the Supervisor's Office and sign in to work with Sally Begay on Tuesday at 1100. Then go to one of the computers that allow you to access the EPR. Open Sally Begay's EPR and review her Admissions Profile. You will learn that she entered the hospital with respiratory distress. The physician's plan is to rule out (R/O) the presence of pneumonia, an infection of the lung tissues. This patient has had chronic lung disease in the form of bronchitis for 10 years, making her susceptible to pneumonia. She also has a history of heart disease.

Now click on **Assessment** and review the trends in physical findings from early Sunday through Tuesday.

1. The assessment of Sally Begay's respirations describes her as "tachypneic." This indicates:
   a. rapid respirations.
   b. irregular respirations.
   c. slow respirations.
   d. normal respirations.

2. The entry for Sally Begay's lung fields on Sunday at 2400 includes the following abbreviation: CR R MB.
   a. What are "crackles"?

 Study Tip: Review physical examination of the thorax and lungs.

3. To determine whether crackles are present in the right middle lobes and base of the lung, the nurse uses what examination technique?
   a. Percussion
   b. Palpation
   c. Auscultation
   d. Inspection

➡ Close the EPR and go inside Room 304 to visit Sally Begay. Click on **Vital Signs** and observe the nurse's technique during measurement of blood pressure and pulse.

4. Which of the following steps did the nurse fail to follow while measuring Sally Begay's blood pressure? (Circle the steps omitted.)

   a. Selecting appropriate size cuff

   b. Ensuring that patient is in correct position

   c. Palpating brachial artery before cuff application

   d. Applying bladder of cuff above artery

   e. Exposing upper arm fully

5. The nurse assesses Sally Begay's radial pulse. Knowing this patient's history, what additional examination would you conduct to assess her cardiac status?

6. Observe the nurse's assessment of Sally Begay's oxygen saturation. Do you expect the oxygen saturation to be accurate? If not, why not?

→ Now review Sally Begay's physical examination. First observe the nurse's examination of the head and neck.

7. When the nurse asks Sally Begay to follow the movement of her fingers, the nurse is assessing:
   a. visual fields.
   b. accommodation.
   c. extraocular movements.
   d. red reflex.

8. To ensure that this examination of the eye is accurate, the nurse must have the patient do what?

9. Considering Sally Begay's presenting clinical condition, what might the nurse expect to find when she palpates the patient's lymph nodes?

10. The nurse demonstrates an excellent technique when assessing Sally Begay's carotid pulse. What is that technique, and why is it important to use?

→ Next, review the examination of Sally Begay's chest and upper extremities.

11. Using the following diagram, show the pattern used by the nurse to auscultate Sally Begay's anterior thorax. Place a **1** at the first site auscultated, followed by a **2** and so on to show the sequence followed.

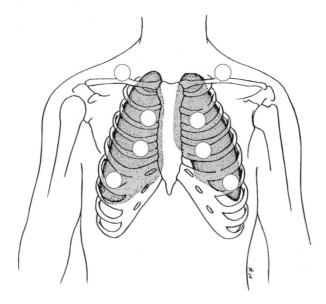

12. List three correct techniques the nurse used as she auscultated over Sally Begay's thorax.

    a.

    b.

    c.

13. Because Sally Begay is being ruled out for the presence of pneumonia, which of the following additional assessments might the nurse have performed while examining the patient's posterior thorax?
    a. Width of costal angle
    b. Tactile fremitus
    c. Location of PMI
    d. Auscultation of adventitious sounds

    Give your rationale for this answer:

14. Sally Begay's Admissions Profile notes that she has had some pain when she coughs. Findings from which of the following examinations performed by the nurse might be affected by this patient's pain?
    a. Chest excursion
    b. Neck range of motion
    c. Abdominal palpation
    d. Heart sounds

→ Now review the examination of Sally Begay's abdomen and lower extremities.

15. On the diagram below, mark with an **X** the locations of where to palpate the following pulses: femoral, popliteal, dorsalis pedis, posterior tibial.

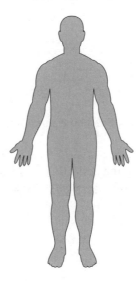

16. Why does the nurse palpate pulses in both extremities at the same time?

17. An abdominal assessment can be very extensive. Provide the rationale for including each of the following in the nursing history for abdominal assessment.

    a. History of abdominal pain:

    b. History of recent weight change:

    c. Patient's normal bowel habits:

    d. History of alcohol ingestion:

→ After reviewing the physical examination, leave the patient's room and go to the Nurses' Station. Find Sally Begay's chart on the bookshelf. (Remember, she is in Room 304.) Open her chart and review the Physical & History, scrolling down to read all pages.

18. Using data from Sally Begay's Physical & History, complete the following assessment categories.

    a. History of abdominal pain?   Yes   No   Not determined

    b. History of recent weight change ? Yes   No   Not determined

    c. Describe patient's normal bowel habits:

    d. History of alcohol ingestion?   Yes   No   Not determined

→ Now click on **Nurses' Notes** and read the nursing plan of care for Sally Begay found in the notes for Saturday.

19. Provide a rationale for giving Sally Begay treatments every 2 hours with an incentive spirometer. Explain how the use of physical assessment techniques can confirm the effects of this treatment. *(Study Tip: Review incentive spirometry in Chapter 39 of your textbook.)*

20. Intermittent positive pressure breathing (IPPB) is a respiratory treatment sometimes administered to improve lung expansion. Why do you think a pain medication was ordered for Sally Begay prior to this treatment?

Exercise 2 – Ira Bradley, Thursday 11:00

 Go to the Supervisor's Office and sign in to work the Thursday 1100 shift with Ira Bradley as your patient. Find out where report is being given on this patient (Room 307). Go to that room and listen to the report.

1. Use the form below to record notes on Ira Bradley's physical status, as given in the nurse's report.

Report Summary:

Diagnosis(es):

Vital Signs: BP _____ RR ____ HR ____ Temp ____ O$_2$ Sat ____

Mental Status:

Lungs/Oxygenation:

Oropharynx:

IV Site:

Lower Extremities:

Now go to one of the computers from which you can access the EPR. Open Ira Bradley's EPR and review his Admissions Profile and assessment data.

2. Which of the following examinations would you prioritize in your own physical assessment of Ira Bradley, based on the nursing report data and the Admissions Profile? (Place an **X** next to all examinations you would prioritize.)

_____ Visual fields

_____ Level of consciousness

_____ Range of motion of extremities

_____ Oral cavity

_____ Lungs

_____ Abdomen

_____ Skin

➡ Go to Room 309 to visit Ira Bradley. Conduct a focused review of his physical examination, observing only the examinations of the head and neck and the chest and upper extremities.

3. What leads the nurse to determine that Ira Bradley has lymphadenopathy?

4. After viewing the examination of Ira Bradley's oral cavity, what would you do differently, and why?

5. On the figure below, place an **X** over each area where the nurse auscultates Ira Bradley's heart sounds.

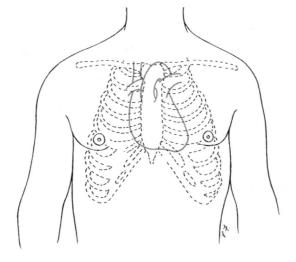

6. Which anatomic site did the nurse *not* auscultate?
   a. PMI
   b. Aortic
   c. Second pulmonic
   d. Pulmonic

7. In Exercise 1 we considered the need to assess tactile fremitus in the case of Sally Begay. Why does the nurse measure tactile fremitus in Ira Bradley's case?
   a. He has a history of substernal pain.
   b. He has tender lymph nodes.
   c. He has had crackles in both lower lung bases.
   d. He has difficulty swallowing.

➡ Leave Ira Bradley's room and return to his EPR. Review his vital signs from Tuesday at 1600 to Wednesday at 1600.

8. Chart Ira Bradley's vital signs on the flow sheet below.

Vital Signs Record/
I/O and Parenteral Fluid Record

Date: _____

HOUR Temp in Centigrade																		
KEY Assume Oral **R**ectal **A**xillary **T**ympanic	42.0 41.5 41.0 40.5 40.0 39.5 39.0 38.5 38.0 37.5 37.0 36.5 36.0 35.5 35.0																	
RESP																		
O$_2$ FLOW																		
O$_2$ SAT																		
BLOOD PRESSURE v Systolic ∧ Diastolic Pulse ●	260 240 220 200 180 160 140 120 100 80 60 40 20																	
REMARKS/TESTING																		

9. Given the information you have, cite three reasons why Ira Bradley is likely to have an increase in heart rate on Wednesday at 1600.

10. Explain why Ira Bradley's temperature dropped to 99.6° F at 2400 on Tuesday.

Communication with the Patient and Health Care Team

/ΟΟ **Reading Assignment:** Communication (Chapter 22)

Patients: Ira Bradley, Room 309
Sally Begay, Room 304

Objectives

- Identify examples of nonverbal communication depicted in the case studies.
- Describe elements of professional communication applied during collection of a nursing history.
- Identify therapeutic communication techniques.
- Critique the nurse's approach during the orientation phase of helping relationships in the case studies.
- Identify factors that create barriers to communication.

Your ability to communicate effectively with patients and their families will influence your ability to provide appropriate nursing care. Talking *with* patients, not *at* patients, can be a difficult skill to learn. Communication requires sensitivity, imagination, active participation, and an astute interpretation of what patients convey through their words and behavior. You must be willing to get to know a patient and to reveal a bit of yourself in order to establish the trust and confidence necessary to communicate therapeutically.

Exercise 1 – Ira Bradley, Thursday 1100

Begin this exercise by going to the Supervisor's Office and signing in to work with Ira Bradley on Thursday at 1100. Then go to Room 307 to listen to the change-of-shift report for this patient. After you have heard the report, proceed to the Nurses' Station, open Ira Bradley's chart, and read the entire Physical & History. (Remember to scroll down to read all pages.) Then read the nurses' notes for Wednesday at 2200.

1. After gathering information about Ira Bradley, identify some challenging communication situations you might face when you meet him.

→ Now it is time to visit Ira Bradley and his wife in Room 309. After entering the room, observe the nurse as she checks the patient's vital signs.

2. When the nurse entered Ira Bradley's room to assess vital signs, which of the following elements of professional communication did she apply? (Circle all correct answers.)

   a. Trustworthiness

   b. Courtesy

   c. Use of name

   d. Privacy and confidentiality

   e. Autonomy and responsibility

   f. Assertiveness

3. What did the nurse do incorrectly when explaining her purpose in needing to check Ira Bradley's vital signs?

→ Now review Ira Bradley's health history. Observe the nurse's assessment in the following categories: Perception/Self-Concept, Role/Relationship, Health Perception, and Coping/Stress.

4. Identify four nonverbal expressions communicated by Ira Bradley and his wife during the nurse's assessment of the Perception/Self-Concept category.

   a.

   b.

   c.

   d.

5. As you review the nurse's assessment, you will notice a number of contextual factors that influence communication between nurse and patient. Match each of the following specific contextual elements from Ira Bradley's health history with the corresponding contextual factor. (A contextual factor may match with more than one contextual element.)

Specific Contextual Element

_____ Ira Bradley is an experienced researcher with advanced education.

_____ Ira Bradley expresses loss of hope.

_____ Ira Bradley suffers from constant fatigue.

_____ Ira Bradley's wife discloses the quality of intimacy between her and her husband.

_____ Nurse initiates conversation to assess Ira Bradley's health status

_____ Ira Bradley and his wife are grieving.

_____ Ira Bradley's wife shares how loss of friends has been difficult.

Contextual Factor

a. Psychophysiologic context

b. Relational context

c. Situational context

d. Environmental context

e. Cultural context

6. Listen again to the nurse as she assesses Ira Bradley and his wife for their perception of stress (found in the Coping/Stress category). Based on their responses to the statement, "Tell me a little bit about the stress in your life," which of the following would be the best follow-up response by the nurse? Explain why.
   a. "Can we provide a comfortable place for you, Mrs. Bradley, to help you get some sleep while you are here?"
   b. "It sounds as though the effects of Mr. Bradley's illness have been very difficult for both of you."
   c. "Your children are important to you; let's talk more about them."
   d. "Don't worry. We will be able to minimize some of the stress you are feeling."

   Give the rationale for your answer:

➤ Now click on **Sexuality/Reproduction** and observe the nurse's assessment of this category of Ira Bradley's health history by selecting each of the three subcategories shown on your screen.

7. During this assessment, the nurse asks Ira Bradley, "Has your tiredness interfered with you and your partner's sexual relations?" This question demonstrates:
   a. focusing.
   b. failure to listen.
   c. changing the subject.
   d. sympathy.

8. Asking questions allows the nurse to gather information necessary for making decisions about a patient's care. Match each of the following nurse's assessment questions with the corresponding type of question.

Nurse's Assessment Question	Type of Question
_____ "So, are you close to your family and your partner?"	a. Open-ended
_____ "How are you feeling about yourself?"	b. Closed-ended
_____ "How do you think about your health?"	
_____ "How about friends? Do you have close friends?"	
_____ "Tell me a little bit about the stress in your life."	

➤ Now click on **Activity** and each of its three subcategories to review this section of Ira Bradley's health history.

9. During the assessment of Occupation/Activity Habits, the nurse asks about the kinds of things Ira Bradley was doing before this last infection. After his response, the nurse asks, "Full- or part-time?" This question is an example of:
   a. summarizing.
   b. focusing.
   c. clarifying.
   d. asking a relevant question.

10. During the assessment of Limitations in ADL, the nurse responds to Ira Bradley, saying, "For example, working at home, helping with chores?" What type of communication technique is the nurse using here? Give the rationale for this type of response.

➤ Review the remaining categories in Ira Bradley's health history.

11. After observing the assessment of Ira Bradley's health history, it is clear that his illness has been very devastating to him. This situation requires a nurse's understanding, empathic response. For each of the following communication techniques, write examples of statements you would use to communicate with Ira Bradley.

Sharing hope:

Sharing empathy:

Summarizing:

Exercise 2 – Sally Begay, Thursday 1100

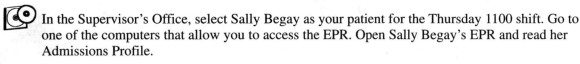 In the Supervisor's Office, select Sally Begay as your patient for the Thursday 1100 shift. Go to one of the computers that allow you to access the EPR. Open Sally Begay's EPR and read her Admissions Profile.

1. As you review the Admissions Profile, identify five interpersonal variables revealed that may influence how Sally Begay will communicate.

    a.

    b.

    c.

    d.

    e.

2. In what way will Sally Begay's difficulty with breathing influence her ability to communicate?

Now go to Room 306 and listen to the change-of-shift report for Sally Begay.

3. Which of the following factors were communicated by the nurse during report? (Circle all correct answers.)

    a. Sally Begay has stable vital signs.

    b. Sally Begay had difficulty sleeping.

    c. Sally Begay is going home today.

    d. Sally Begay will require discharge teaching.

    e. Sally Begay had respiratory complications during the night.

After listening to report, proceed to Room 304. Go inside and observe the nurse's introduction prior to measuring Sally Begay's vital signs.

4. Write a description of how you would greet Sally Begay prior to measuring her vital signs.

→ Now click on **Health History** and review the nurse's assessment of the Perception/Self-Concept category.

5. The nurse asks the question, "How are you feeling about yourself?" This is an example of:
   a. an open-ended question.
   b. a closed-ended question.

6. When the nurse asks Sally Begay whether she has any worries or concerns, the patient says she is worried about things at home and also for the animals being cared for at home. Write an example of an open-ended question that would clarify Sally Begay's response.

7. While assessing the Perception of Abilities category, the nurse asks Sally Begay how she will care for herself when she returns home. After listening to the patient's response, what is the best therapeutic approach for the nurse to take in order to better understand how Sally Begay will care for herself?
   a. Confronting
   b. Self-disclosing
   c. Paraphrasing
   d. Asking for explanation

→ Return to Room 306 to observe the health team meeting on Sally Begay. After listening to the team meeting, go to the Nurses' Station. Open Sally Begay's chart, click on **Health Team**, and read the summary notes from each of the health team members.

8. The health team meeting is an example of:
   a. communication in a public zone.
   b. communication in a social zone.
   c. communication in an intimate zone.
   d. communication in a personal zone.

9. In her report, the social worker identifies four main points of concern. One is her concern about cultural sensitivity in providing resources and education to Sally Begay. What information did you learn from the Admissions Profile (question 1) that might be helpful regarding this issue?

10. As the nurse caring for Sally Begay, write an example of how you might explain to her the ending of your nurse-patient relationship.

Exercise 3

1. Consider this question: Which patient would you prefer to communicate with—Ira Bradley or Sally Begay? Write a one- to two-page summary explaining your decision. Defend your explanation by addressing the following: your past experiences with communicating in challenging situations, any perceptual biases you might have, and the effect your patient's values, health status and emotions have on your ability to communicate.

Patient Education in Practice

Reading Assignment: Patient Education (Chapter 23)

Patients: Carmen Gonzales, Room 302
Andrea Wang, Room 310

Objectives

- Identify domains of learning as they apply to the learning needs of patients in the case studies.
- Determine factors that influence patients' motivation and ability to learn.
- Identify resources for learning.
- Write a learning objective correctly.
- Develop a teaching plan for patients in the case studies.
- Select appropriate teaching methods based on a patient's learning needs.
- Describe approaches to evaluate a patient's success at learning.

As a nurse you will have numerous opportunities to educate patients and their families on ways to manage their health care needs and to promote their level of health. Education is an important part of your role. Patients and families have the right to information that allows them to make intelligent, informed decisions about their health and lifestyle. In the acute care setting, patients are discharged home as soon as possible, making timely patient education even more essential. Integrating education into all of your nursing care approaches is very important. For example, you can educate while administering medications to a patient, bathing a patient, assisting a patient during a meal, and ambulating a patient down the hall. Making education relevant, timely, and even fun enhances a patient's ability to learn. To be an effective educator, you must accurately identify a patient's learning needs, consider the patient's willingness and ability to learn, and then select the most effective teaching strategies.

Exercise 1 – Carmen Gonzales, Tuesday 1100

Begin by signing in on the desktop computer in the Supervisor's Office. Select Carmen Gonzales as your patient for the Tuesday 1100 shift. Then go to one of the computers from which you can access the EPR. Open Carmen Gonzales' EPR and review her Admissions Profile.

1. Patient education begins with a thorough nursing assessment. After reviewing Carmen Gonzales' Admissions Profile, identify factors from her history for each of the following learning assessment categories.

   a. Learning needs:

   b. Motivation to learn:

   c. Ability to learn:

➤ Close the EPR and proceed to the Nurses' Station. Open Carmen Gonzales' chart and review her Physical & History. (Remember to scroll down to read all pages.)

2. What information from the Physical & History suggests that Carmen Gonzales might have difficulty with motivation or ability to learn?

3. List three potential resources for Carmen Gonzales' learning.

➤ Before you visit Carmen Gonzales, go to Room 306 and listen to the change-of-shift report given by the nurse who worked with her earlier this morning.

4. The change-of-shift report revealed Carmen Gonzales' clinical status during the night and through this morning. Her responsiveness to your continued assessment will likely be influenced by which of the following?
   a. Wound status
   b. Reduction in pain
   c. Increase in blood pressure
   d. Lung congestion

→ Now proceed to Carmen Gonzales' room (302). Once inside, review her entire health history.

5. Match each of the following findings identified from Carmen Gonzales' health history with the corresponding learning principle. (A learning principle may apply to more than one finding.)

Learning Principle	Health History Finding
_____ Motivation to learn	a. "I can't do anything without feeling tired."
_____ Ability to learn	b. "I don't have a family doctor. I don't do checkups very often."
_____ Resources for learning	c. "We are accustomed to eating a certain way."
_____ Learning needs	d. Patient agrees to work with nurse or other health care providers on a teaching plan.
	e. "I see things a bit fuzzy."
	f. "My daughter will be with us."
	g. "I don't feel well. I feel a bit helpless."

6. Carmen Gonzales' Physical & History indicates that she received education on diabetes 5 months ago. However, in the health history she tells the nurse that she and her husband are accustomed to eating a certain way. Her diet history reveals that her diet is fairly high in carbohydrates. In which of the following learning domains will Carmen Gonzales likely require instruction?
   a. Cognitive learning
   b. Affective learning
   c. Psychomotor learning

7. Diabetes education can include a number of different topics. Match each of the following learning topics with the corresponding learning domain. (A learning domain may apply to more than one learning topic.)

Learning Topic	Learning Domain
_____ Preparing insulin in a syringe	a. Affective learning
_____ Planning an 1800-calorie diabetic diet including appropriate food preferences	b. Cognitive learning
_____ Knowing side effects of insulin	c. Psychomotor learning
_____ Self-administering insulin	
_____ Adopting a plan with her husband that includes daily exercise	
_____ Performing routine inspection of condition of her feet.	

8. Review your assessment findings to begin developing a nursing diagnosis for Carmen Gonzales. Read the following lists of defining characteristics for two possible nursing diagnoses: Ineffective health maintenance and Knowledge deficit. Place an **X** next to all those that apply to Carmen Gonzales.

Ineffective Health Maintenance	**Knowledge Deficit**
_____ Demonstrates lack of knowledge regarding basic health practices	_____ Verbalizes lack of knowledge
_____ Reports or observed inability to take responsibility for meeting basic health practices	_____ Inaccurate follow-through on instruction
_____ History of lack of health-seeking behavior	_____ Inaccurate performance of test
_____ Expressed interest in improving health behavior	_____ Inappropriate or exaggerated behaviors (e.g., hostility/agitation)
_____ Lack of equipment/financial/other resources	
_____ Impairment of personal support systems	

9. Which of the two nursing diagnoses from question 8 is most appropriate for Carmen Gonzales, based on what you know about her at this time? Explain your decision.

10. In developing a teaching plan of care for Carmen Gonzales, it is important to develop learning objectives. Which of the following is a correctly worded learning objective?
   a. Patient will identify a meal plan for a 24-hour period that includes foods allowed within an 1800-calorie diabetic diet by day of discharge.
   b. Patient will understand the importance of proper foods to eat within an 1800-calorie diabetic diet to achieve blood glucose control.
   c. Patient will identify a meal plan that includes foods allowed within an 1800-calorie diabetic diet.
   d. Patient will prepare foods and identify food sources allowed within an 1800-calorie diabetic diet by day of discharge.

11. From your assessment of Carmen Gonzales, you understand that her clinical status makes it important for you to consider the timing of teaching sessions. Describe how your teaching plan would address timing.

12. Diabetic patients can potentially be instructed on a variety of topics. From what you know about Carmen Gonzales, identify the top three priorities to consider in a teaching plan.

_____ Administration of insulin

_____ Development of a meal plan within calorie restrictions

_____ Methods for performing routine foot care

_____ Side effects of hypoglycemia

_____ Blood glucose monitoring at home

_____ Sick-day management

_____ Physiology of diabetes and how it affects her blood sugar level

13. Develop a teaching plan for Carmen Gonzales, based on the nursing diagnosis of Ineffective health maintenance and the three priorities identified in question 12.

Nursing Diagnosis: Ineffective health maintenance

Goals   **Expected Outcomes**

Interventions   **Rationale**

Evaluation

14. A variety of instructional methods can be used when teaching patients. If your teaching topic was diabetic foot care, which of the following instructional methods might work best?
    a. Group instruction
    b. Role playing
    c. Demonstration
    d. Use of printed material

15. What have you learned from Carmen Gonzales' history that might limit the use of printed material?

16. Which of the following instructional methods might work best in helping Carmen Gonzales develop a meal plan?
    a. Role playing
    b. Analogies
    c. Discovery
    d. Demonstration

17. Match each of the following learning behaviors with the best evaluation approach.

Learning Behavior	Evaluation Approach
_____ Adhering to a diet for 7 days	a. Asking questions
_____ Identifying symptoms of insulin reaction	b. Self-reporting
_____ Measuring blood glucose	c. Demonstration

Exercise 2 – Andrea Wang, Thursday 1100

 Return to the Supervisor's Office. This time, sign in to work with Andrea Wang on Thursday at 1100. Proceed to Room 307 to hear the change-of-shift report. Then go to the Nurses' Station and open Andrea Wang's chart. Read the Physical & History and the nurses' notes.

1. When you compare Andrea Wang with Carmen Gonzales in Exercise 1, you will quickly recognize that Carmen Gonzales is dealing with chronic disease processes, whereas Andrea Wang is faced with an acute, life-changing injury. As a result, what learning principle is most important to consider as you plan to assess Andrea Wang's learning needs?
    a. Active participation
    b. Ability to learn
    c. Psychosocial adaptation to illness
    d. Physical capability

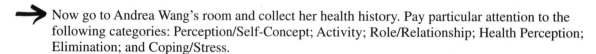 Now go to Andrea Wang's room and collect her health history. Pay particular attention to the following categories: Perception/Self-Concept; Activity; Role/Relationship; Health Perception; Elimination; and Coping/Stress.

2. Based on your assessment, match each of the following stages of psychosocial adaptation with Andrea Wang's corresponding behavior.

Behavior	Psychosocial Adaptation
_____ Does not want to discuss incontinence.	a. Bargaining
_____ Says, "I can't believe this has happened."	b. Anger
_____ Says, "I hope I'll have some movement."	c. Denial

3. A colleague recommends that you begin to talk to Andrea Wang about making adjustments within the home to accommodate a wheelchair. What would be your response? Give your rationale.

4. Andrea Wang explains in her health perception assessment that she likes to talk things out when learning new things. This suggests that an appropriate teaching approach might be:
    a. use of printed material.
    b. analogies.
    c. discovery.
    d. use of computer instruction.

The health care team plays a valuable role in planning patient instruction. Go to the health team meeting in Room 308 and listen to each member's report. Then go to the Nurses' Station and read their written reports by clicking on **Health Team** in Andrea Wang's chart.

5. The case manager has concerns about family support for Andrea Wang. Identify two teaching approaches that might be effective ways to involve the family.

7

Documentation Principles

⟱ **Reading Assignment:** Documentation (Chapter 24)

Patients: David Ruskin, Room 303
Sally Begay, Room 304

Objectives

- Identify elements of quality documentation in written records and verbal reports.
- Explain the relationship between documented information and the nurse's responsibility for follow-up care.
- Write a nursing progress note.
- Critique a change-of-shift report.
- Explain the type of information to be communicated when a change in a patient's condition occurs.

Documentation of patient care must be accurate and timely to ensure continuity of care. Good documentation means good communication. As a nurse you will be responsible for conveying to other nurses and health care professionals your patient's condition and needs, your interventions, and the patient's responses to care. Using the guidelines for quality documentation and reporting ensures that efficient, individualized care will be delivered to your patient.

Exercises within this lesson will allow you to identify the principles used in documenting care of the patients in the case studies. You will be able to critique whether nurses in the case studies communicated information about patient care in a comprehensive and accurate manner.

Exercise 1 – David Ruskin, Tuesday 0700

 In the Supervisor's Office sign in to work with David Ruskin on Tuesday at 0700. Then proceed to Room 307 to hear the nurse's change-of-shift report for this patient.

1. Use the form below to take notes during the change-of-shift report.

Patient's Name: Admitted:

Diagnosis(es):

Vital Signs: BP _____ RR ____ HR ____ Temp ____ O_2 Sat ____

Lungs:

Heart:

IV:

Other:

---

2. A good report should direct you in the care of your patient. Match each of the following elements of David Ruskin's report with the corresponding actions you should take.

Report Elements

_____ Some pain in left arm and side

_____ IV in left hand

_____ Hurts some to breathe

_____ All peripheral pulses palpable and extremities warm

_____ Abrasions along left side with no signs of infection

Actions

a. Check for depth of breathing; measure chest excursion.

b. Inspect leg and trunk for condition of skin.

c. Palpate pulses of upper and lower extremities.

d. Inspect condition of IV site in hand.

e. Ask patient to identify location of pain and to rate intensity.

➡️ Now go to David Ruskin's room (303). Enter the room, click on **Physical**, and review the nurse's physical assessment. Also observe the assessment of the patient's pain by clicking first on **Vital Signs**, then on **Pain Rating**.

3. Based on what you observed, record the nurse's findings for each of the following recommended actions.

    a. Check for depth of breathing; measure chest excursion:

    b. Inspect leg and trunk for condition of skin:

    c. Palpate pulses of upper and lower extremities:

    d. Inspect condition of IV in hand:

    e. Ask patient to identify location of pain and to rate intensity:

4. Compare the data from the nurse's change-of-shift report with your observation of the nurse's assessment of David Ruskin.

    a. What information in the report do you think is likely to be inaccurate?

    b. What would you do to clarify this problem?

➡️ Exit the patient's room and go to the bookshelf in the Nurses' Station. Open David Ruskin's chart and review the Physical & History and the nurses' notes. (Remember to scroll down to read all the pages.)

5. Mark on the clock face below the time (in **standard time**) when David Ruskin was admitted to the nursing unit from postanesthesia. Then mark the time (in **standard time**) when the first nurses' note was written.

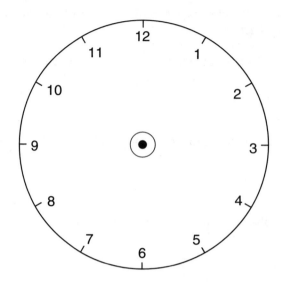

6. Part of the nurses' note for Sunday 2030 provides objective data for David Ruskin. Rewrite that portion of the note so that it is more organized.

7. Read the nurses' note written for Monday at 1615. Give special attention to the analysis and assessment section.

   a. What time (in standard time) was the note entered?

   b. After reading the analysis section, explain why the note is incomplete.

8. Read the nurses' note written for Wednesday at 1300. Rewrite the SOAP note as a DAR note.

D:

A:

R:

➜ Exit the chart and click on the computer to the right of the bookshelf to access the EPR. Open David Ruskin's EPR and review his assessment records for the period of Sunday 2000 through Monday 0800.

9. As you review David Ruskin's assessment data, which of the following assessment findings alert the nurse that something out of the ordinary has been observed or has occurred, requiring the nurse's follow-up? (Circle all correct answers.)

a. Speech

b. Edema

c. Pupils

d. Movement

e. Blood pressure

10. What charting system is used to make it easy for nurses to reduce repetitive recording of normal findings?

Exercise 2 – Sally Begay, Tuesday 0700

 Go to the Supervisor's Office and sign in to work the Tuesday 0700 shift with Sally Begay as your patient. Then go to one of the computers that allow you to access the EPR. Open Sally Begay's EPR and review her Admissions Profile, as well as her vital signs and assessment data.

1. An EPR can tell a story. As you review Sally Begay's data, complete the flow chart below. (*Note: Not all time periods shown in the EPR are included here.*)

Day/Time	Sat admit	Sat 2000	Sun 0800	Sun 1600	Sun 2400	Mon 0800	Mon 1600	Mon 2000	Mon 2400
Temp									
BP									
HR									
RR									
O_2 Sat									
Pain									

Admission diagnoses:

Significant past history:

From the assessment data, identify four criteria to be concerned about, knowing Sally Begay has pneumonia:

2. As you review the chart you completed in question 1, match each of the following vital sign values with the corresponding clinical trend revealed in the chart. (More than one vital sign value will apply to each clinical trend.)

Vital Sign Value	Clinical Trend
_____ Temperature	a. Condition stable
_____ Heart rate	b. Condition improves
_____ Respirations	c. Condition unstable
_____ Blood pressure	
_____ Oxygen saturation	
_____ Pain	

→ Exit the EPR and go to the Nurses' Station. Open Sally Begay's chart and review the nurses' notes for Saturday at 2100, Sunday at 1400, and Monday at 1300.

3. What does the nurses' note for Saturday fail to describe with regard to Sally Begay's chest pain and lung sounds?

4. The plan of care in the nurses' notes for Saturday recommends oxygen by nasal cannula. In what way does Sally Begay respond to this therapy by Sunday?

5. If you were to change the nurses' note for Sunday, how would you write the description about the pain medication to make it more complete?

6. Write the nurses' note for Monday at 1300 in a PIE format.

P:

I:

E:

➡ Read the nurses' notes for Monday at 2200. Then close the chart and go to the room where the change-of-shift report is being given for Sally Begay. (Remember: You can find this by going to the bulletin board in the Nurses' Station or by moving your cursor across the animated map.)

7. Answer the following questions from the information heard in the report:

a. What is the oxygen saturation on room air?

b. What is the oxygen saturation on 2 liters of oxygen?

c. Compared with Monday at 2200, did Sally Begay's temperature increase or decrease during the night?

d. Since Sally Begay has been eating less than 50% of her meals, why did the nurse not report her response to the plan for eating snacks?

LESSON 8

Safe Medication Administration in Practice

 Reading Assignment: Medication Administration (Chapter 34)

Patients: David Ruskin, Room 303
Carmen Gonzales, Room 302

Study Tip: Have your pharmacology book close by as you complete this lesson.

Objectives

- Explain the rationale for the selection of specific medications for patients in the case studies.
- Explain the rationale for why certain medication routes are chosen for patients in the case studies.
- Identify types of medication actions.
- Perform medication dosage calculations.
- Describe process for correct administration of medication.
- Explain nursing implications for administering medications.
- Discuss common sources of medication errors.
- Explain factors that will influence patients' ability to self-administer medications.

Pharmacologic therapy is common for patients with acute and chronic health care problems. Because medications can cause a variety of actions—many of which are nontherapeutic—the safe administration of medications is critical. You can never be too cautious in administering medications. Always know what medication your patient has been prescribed and why. Know each medication, its purpose, therapeutic action, and common side effects. Be aware of the basic principles used to calculate and prepare medications safely and accurately. Know the effects that medications may have on your patient's behavior and physical condition so that you can properly monitor the patient and evaluate whether the drugs have been effective.

Patient education is an important part of drug therapy. It is your responsibility as a nurse to be sure patients know how to self-administer medications safely. This means that patients must know the reason for receiving each medication and how it will affect them physically, cognitively, and behaviorally. Unless patients know the side effects that warn of an inappropriate drug response, they may not consult their health care provider when problems arise. Home environments and daily routines influence how patients take their medications. It is important that you actively problem-solve with patients and families by anticipating possible barriers to safe medication administration in the home and workplace.

Exercise 1 – David Ruskin, Tuesday 1100

 In the Supervisor's Office sign in to work with David Ruskin on Tuesday at 1100. Go to the Nurses' Station, open David Ruskin's chart, and read his Physical & History. (Remember to scroll down to read all pages.) Close his chart and go to the blue notebook that contains the medication administration record (MAR). Open David Ruskin's MAR and review the medications currently ordered for him.

1. List David Ruskin's allergies.

2. David Ruskin is receiving cefoxitin, 1 g IVPB q6h to:
   a. control or relieve pain caused by fracture and abrasions.
   b. prevent development of infection from injury to soft tissues and bone.
   c. improve ventilation affected by chest pain.
   d. prevent cerebral edema from closed head injury.

3. According to the MAR, David Ruskin's last dose of cefoxitin was given at 1500. His next dose is due at:
   a. 2100.
   b. 2200.
   c. 1900.
   d. 2000.

4. Explain David Ruskin's order for oxycodone by answering the following questions:

   a. What is the maximum dose he can receive at any one time?

   b. Once a dose has been given, when is the earliest he can receive the next dose?

   c. What does a PRN order mean?

 Study Tip: Review Chapter 42 for pros and cons of PRN orders for analgesia.

 Now return to the Nurses' Station. Open David Ruskin's chart and read the expired MAR report. This report reviews the medications he received Sunday through Monday. After reviewing these, exit the chart and go to the computer on the counter below the bookshelf. Open David Ruskin's EPR and review his vital sign data, specifically his pain acuity scores.

5. Between Monday and Tuesday, David Ruskin's analgesic order changed from ketorolac, 30 mg IM, to oxycodone, 5 to 10 mg PO. Can you explain why?

6. The order for ketorolac is 30 mg IM. The medication comes in 15 mg per ml. Use the basic formula below to calculate the volume of medication you would administer to David Ruskin.

$$\frac{\text{Dose ordered}}{\text{Dose on hand}} \text{ x Amount on hand } = \text{Amount to administer}$$

7. The reason for administering cefoxitin by IV piggy back to David Ruskin is to:
   a. maintain a constant therapeutic blood level of antibiotic.
   b. dilute the irritating antibiotic in a large volume of fluid.
   c. administer the drug in a single concentrated dose.
   d. minimize David Ruskin's fluid intake during drug administration.

→ Now return to the sign-in computer in the Supervisor's Office. Keep David Ruskin as your patient, but change your shift to Tuesday 0700. Now go to David Ruskin's room, click on **Vital Signs**, and observe the nurse's assessment of the patient's pain rating. Next, review the physical examination. Finally, click on **Medications** and observe the nurse as she administers medications to the patient.

8. As you observe the nurse caring for David Ruskin, what did she do to ensure the right patient would receive the right medication?

9. What did the nurse fail to do as she prepared to give the medication?

10. Numerous factors influence the choice of route for medication administration. Match each of the following routes with its corresponding characteristics. (More than one characteristic may match with each route.)

Characteristic	Route
_____ Creates anxiety for patient	a. Oral
_____ Cannot be given when patient has gastric suction	b. Parenteral
_____ Creates a risk for introducing infection	c. Topical
_____ Provides mainly a local effect	
_____ Is convenient and economical	
_____ Results in rapid absorption	

11. After receiving a dose of oxycodone, David Ruskin would probably exhibit some physical and behavioral changes. Which of the following changes would you expect to see during your evaluation? (Place an **X** next to all correct answers.)

_____ He moves more slowly in bed.

_____ His pain acuity score falls.

_____ He grimaces less when sitting up.

_____ His heart rate may increase.

_____ His pain acuity score rises.

_____ The pain along his rib cage decreases.

Exercise 2 – Carmen Gonzales, Thursday 0700

 Return to the Supervisor's Office and sign in to work with Carmen Gonzales on Thursday at 0700. Go to the Nurses' Station and open her chart. First check the physician's orders to see which medications Carmen Gonzales is currently taking. Then review her Physical & History.

1. Carmen Gonzales is receiving a variety of medications. Match each of the following medications with the corresponding purpose for which she is receiving that medication.

Medication	Purpose
_____ Glyburide	a. Hormone for control of blood sugar levels above 150 mg/dl
_____ Oxycodone	b. Antibiotic to treat infection of soft tissue
_____ Furosemide	c. Diuretic to treat congestive heart failure and hypertension
_____ Insulin	d. Oral hypoglycemic for treating type 2 diabetes
_____ Cefoxitin	e. Opioid analgesic for pain in soft tissues

→ Close the patient's chart and go to the computer under the bookshelf. Access Carmen Gonzales'
EPR and review her assessment findings for Wednesday.

2. The regular administration of furosemide should influence which of the following physical
   findings noted in Carmen Gonzales' EPR?
   a. Pain in leg and level of fatigue
   b. Level of edema and lung field congestion
   c. Blood sugar and orientation
   d. Blood pressure and wound drainage

3. Carmen Gonzales turns on her nurse call light. When you enter her room, she tells you that
   she has a rash over her abdomen and arms. Her skin itches. This is most likely the result of:
   a. a side effect.
   b. a therapeutic effect.
   c. an idiosyncratic effect.
   d. an allergic reaction.

4. Which medication do you think is most likely the cause of Carmen Gonzales' rash?

→ Close the EPR and go to Carmen Gonzales' room (302). Once inside, observe the nurse as he
administers medication to the patient.

5. What action did the nurse take to ensure Carmen Gonzales received the right medications?

6. How soon should the nurse return to evaluate Carmen Gonzales' response after administering the oral medications?
   a. 60 minutes
   b. 30 minutes
   c. 15 minutes
   d. 10 minutes

7. Among the medications Carmen Gonzales is receiving, which can create a more rapid
   response? Explain why.

8. Acetaminophen, 650 mg PO, is ordered q4h for mild pain. When you go to the medication room, you find that acetaminophen tablets are available in grains only. What must you do in order to administer the medication?

9. Carmen Gonzales' EPR reveals that she is receiving incremental doses of insulin when her blood glucose is above 150 mg/dl. In preparing to administer insulin to this patient, you remember that:
   a. only regular insulin is used in a sliding scale.
   b. insulin is administered in milligrams.
   c. you should administer the insulin injection in a different anatomic site each time.
   d. you should insert the syringe needle into tissues at a 15-degree angle.

LESSON 9

Comfort

Reading Assignment: Comfort (Chapter 42)
Patients: David Ruskin, Room 303
Carmen Gonzales, Room 302

Objectives

- Identify the rationale for the physical assessment measures a nurse selects when a patient has pain.
- Explain the physiologic responses to expect when a patient has pain.
- Identify nonverbal responses to pain.
- Describe how to apply critical thinking during assessment of patients who experience pain.
- Describe potential nursing interventions for relieving pain of patients in the case studies.

You have already learned that pain is the most common reason people seek health care. Your ability as a nurse to provide comfort for your patients requires being willing to accept and understand their pain experience. Comfort is a basic patient need. Basic to successful nursing practice is the ability to select the appropriate measures to help relieve pain and enable patients to live a more productive and satisfying life. The exercises contained within this lesson will improve your ability to assess pain and to understand how to select nursing interventions on the basis of an individual patient's pain response.

Exercise 1 – David Ruskin, Thursday 1100

In the Supervisor's Office, sign in on the desktop computer. Select Thursday 1100 as your shift and David Ruskin as your patient. Go to the mobile computer in the hallway, outside the Supervisor's Office, and access David Ruskin's EPR. First click on **Admissions** and read the Admissions Profile thoroughly. Then review the vital signs data, paying particular attention to David Ruskin's pain ratings from Monday through Wednesday. The clinical information you review provides a knowledge base that will allow you to critically think and anticipate David Ruskin's needs.

1. Identify the potential sources and corresponding locations of injury that may cause pain for David Ruskin.

   Source   **Location**

2. How would you rate the quality of the description of David Ruskin's injuries in the Admissions Profile? What would you do to improve the description?

→ Now click on **Assessment** in the EPR and review David Ruskin's data for Monday.

3. Knowing the source and location of this patient's injuries, in addition to the findings from his Admissions Profile, which of the following areas do you expect to be affected by his pain? (Place an **X** next to all areas that apply.)

   _____ Sleep

   _____ Speech

   _____ Mobility

   _____ Abdomen

   _____ Chest expansion

   _____ Respiratory pattern

4. Pain can result in stimulation of the sympathetic nervous system. For each of the following vital signs, indicate the type of response you would expect from acute pain by marking with ↑, ↓, or **no change**.

   _____ Heart rate

   _____ Respirations

   _____ Blood pressure

➡ Return to the vital signs section of David Ruskin's EPR. Review his vital signs for Wednesday at 1600. Then check his Admission Profile for Sunday at 1600 and review his vital signs at that time.

5. As you compare David Ruskin's baseline on Wednesday with that on Sunday, indicate the type of response he experienced (↑, ↓, or **no change**) for each of the following vital signs.

_____ Heart rate

_____ Respirations

_____ Blood pressure

Explain the reason for your findings:

➡ Close the EPR and go to the Nurses' Station. Open David Ruskin's chart (Room 303) and review the expired MARs from Sunday through Wednesday. This summarizes medications he has received since his admission.

6. Describe the nursing principles for administering analgesics that were followed in David Ruskin's case.

7. Describe the nursing principles for administering analgesics that were *not* followed in David Ruskin's case.

➡ Now that you have had time to learn quite a bit about David Ruskin's condition, go to Room 303 to visit him.

8. Consider what you have learned about David Ruskin's condition from his chart and the EPR. To assess more closely the extent of his injuries, explain how you would adapt your physical examination in the following three areas.

a. Head and neck:

b. Chest and upper extremities:

c. Abdomen and lower extremities:

Study Tip: Review condition of scalp and skin and musculoskeletal examination in Chapter 32 in your textbook.

→ Inside David Ruskin's room, click on **Physical** and observe the nurse performing each component of the physical examination.

9. Why does the nurse ask David Ruskin whether he has discomfort when he turns his neck?

10. Why does the nurse check for chest excursion?

11. What did the nurse overlook when examining the upper and lower extremities?

→ Now observe the patient closely as the nurse asks him to sit up for the chest examination.

12. Identify three nonverbal behaviors David Ruskin uses to express his pain.

a.

b.

c.

13. The characteristics of a patient's pain help you as a nurse to plan interventions that may bring pain relief. Which of the following characteristics of David Ruskin's pain have you been able to determine after reviewing his chart, EPR, and physical examination? (Place an **X** next to all that apply.)

_____ Onset and duration

_____ Location

_____ Intensity

_____ Quality

_____ Pain pattern

_____ Relief measures

_____ Concomitant symptoms

➡ It is also important to include in your assessment database a review of how pain is affecting David Ruskin's activities of daily living and the expectations he has of how pain might affect him once he returns home. To accomplish this, click on **Health History** and observe the interview in each of the 12 categories.

14. Identify four areas of the health history that indicate the effects of pain on David Ruskin.

a.

b.

c.

d.

15. Given what you now know about David Ruskin, consider the knowledge you might criti-cally apply in your development of a nursing care plan. Explain how each of the following knowledge areas will help you in developing a plan of care.

    a. Culture:

    b. Nonpharmacologic pain therapies:

    c. Caring in families:

16. Identify two nonpharmacologic pain relief measures you believe would be effective for David Ruskin, and give a rationale. Make your rationale specific to what you know about David Ruskin.

Exercise 2 – Carmen Gonzales, Thursday 1100

 Return to the Supervisor's Office (Room 301) and sign in to work with Carmen Gonzales on Thursday at 1100. Then go to one of the computers that allow you to access the EPR. In this exercise you will further explore pain assessment and make some comparisons between David Ruskin's pain and the pain experienced by another patient, Carmen Gonzales. Open Carmen Gonzales' EPR and read the Admissions Profile, the assessment flow sheet, and the vital signs flow sheet.

1. Based on what you have learned, complete the following worksheet.

Admission Diagnosis:

Admission Vital Signs: BP _____ RR _____ HR _____ Overweight __ Underweight __

Effects of Pain (check all that apply):

Trouble sleeping ____   Changes in elimination ____

Limited ability to perform   Restricted mobility ____
  instrumental ADL ____

Reduced chest excursion ____   Behavioral changes ____

Pain Intensity Rating:

Time of Assessment	Admit	Mon 1200	Mon 1600	Mon 2000	Mon 2400	Tues 1600	Tues 2000	Tues 2400
Pain Rating								

---

2. In the EPR, what concomitant pain symptoms were reported for Carmen Gonzales? Is there any explanation for these symptoms other than pain?

3. Both Carmen Gonzales and David Ruskin have acute pain. Indicate whether each of the following statements describing acute pain is true or false.

   a. T F Acute pain has a rapid onset usually lasting less than 6 months.

   b. T F Health care providers are usually less willing to treat acute pain than chronic pain.

   c. T F The cause for acute pain is usually unknown.

   d. T F Acute pain can threaten a patient's psychologic progress

→ Close the EPR and go to the Nurses' Station. Open Carmen Gonzales' chart (Room 302) and review the expired MARs.

4. As you read the order for morphine sulfate, 2–5 mg q1–2h PRN and you review the patient's pain intensity ratings from Monday to Tuesday, what problem do you find in Carmen Gonzales' therapy? What might you consider as an alternative to the way the morphine sulfate is ordered?

→ Now close the chart and go inside Room 302 to visit Carmen Gonzales. Click on **Physical** and review the physical examination of her abdomen and lower extremities. Pay close attention to the nurse's assessment of the lower extremities.

5. If you had examined Carmen Gonzales, how would you have assessed the pain in her left lower leg differently?

→ Now review the patient's health history interview. Pay particular attention to the assessment of the following categories: Perception/Self-Concept, Activity, and Sleep-Rest.

6. Now that you have a more thorough view of Carmen Gonzales' health status, explain how her fear of not walking again, her inactivity, and her lack of sleep may influence her perception of pain.

7. Which one of the following factors is most likely to influence the meaning that pain has for Carmen Gonzales?
   a. Her catholic religion
   b. Her husband's retirement
   c. Her cultural background
   d. Her experience of having diabetes

LESSON 10

Oxygenation

/OꙨ **Reading Assignment:** Oxygenation (Chapter 39)

Patients: Sally Begay, Room 304
            David Ruskin, Room 303
            Andrea Wang, Room 310

Objectives

- Identify relationship of cardiac and respiratory alterations.
- Identify how the respiratory and cardiac conditions of patients in the case studies influence ventilation and respiration.
- Describe factors that influence oxygenation.
- Assess the oxygenation status of patients in the case studies.
- Apply critical thinking in care of patients with cardiopulmonary alterations.
- Discuss rationale for use of clinical interventions for patients in the case studies.
- Evaluate effect of interventions used in the case studies.

The cardiac and respiratory systems function together to supply the body's oxygen demands. The function of the cardiac system is to deliver oxygen, nutrients, and other substances to the tissues and to remove the waste products of cellular metabolism through the cardiac pump, vascular system, and integration of the respiratory, digestive, and renal systems. Through ventilation, perfusion, and diffusion, the respiratory system exchanges gases between the environmental air and the blood. When a dysfunction of the cardiopulmonary system exists, the patient may experience any number of signs and symptoms. The patient's lifestyle, the environment, and the effects of medications and other therapies further complicate how a patient reacts. As a nurse you must be able to astutely assess changes in a patient's condition and recognize when intervention is necessary to restore a patient's oxygenation status. Critical thinking becomes especially important because of the complexity of some cardiopulmonary alterations.

Exercise 1 – Sally Begay, Tuesday 1100

 Sign in on the desktop computer in the Supervisor's Office (Room 301). Select Sally Begay as your patient for the Tuesday 1100 shift. Proceed to the Nurses' Station and open her chart (304) Read the Physical & History carefully. (Remember to scroll down to read all pages.) Then review the physicians' notes.

Study Tip: Review the physiology of pneumonia in a reference book.

1. Sally Begay's initial diagnosis of pneumonia is a condition that affects which of the following structures of the lung?
   a. Respiratory muscles
   b. Pleural space
   c. Bronchi
   d. Alveoli

2. Because of inflammation of the alveoli, Sally Begay is most likely to have an alteration of:
   a. pulmonary circulation.
   b. diffusion.
   c. work of breathing.
   d. regulation of respiration.

3. Sally Begay's 10-year history of chronic bronchitis is a complicating factor. Chronic bronchitis results in an excessive secretion of mucus in the bronchi, thus causing an alteration in:
   a. compliance.
   b. elastic recoil of lung.
   c. airway resistance.
   d. diffusion.

4. Sally Begay presents with a number of symptoms. Match each of the following symptoms with its corresponding description.

Symptom	Description
_____ Chest pain	a. Clinical sign of hypoxia, manifested by feeling of breathlessness
_____ Dyspnea	
_____ Fatigue	b. Subjective sensation of patient reporting loss of endurance
_____ Productive cough	c. Condition in which patient must sit or raise head on multiple pillows to breathe
_____ Orthopnea	
	d. Sputum material coughed up from the lungs
	e. Subjective symptom worsened by coughing

5. If Sally Begay were able to expectorate mucous following her cough, you would expect it to be:
   a. clear and watery.
   b. yellow or green with a foul odor.
   c. red and tenacious.
   d. white and frothy.

6. Do you believe that Sally Begay was experiencing hypoxia when she was admitted to the hospital? Defend your answer.

7. The Physical & History revealed that Sally Begay's PMI was found to be slightly to the left of the midline. What does this indicate? *(Study Tip: Review cardiopulmonary assessment in Chapter 32 in your textbook.)*

➡ Close the patient's chart and access the MAR (the blue notebook on the counter). Review Sally Begay's currently ordered medications.

8. Refer to a pharmacology reference and explain why Sally Begay is receiving the following medications.

   a. Digoxin:

   b. Hydrochlorothiazide:

   c. Erythromycin:

➡ Now proceed to Room 304 to visit Sally Begay. Begin by reviewing her physical examination. Pay particular attention to findings during the head and neck and chest/upper extremity examinations. *(Study Tip: Review cardiopulmonary assessment in Chapter 32 in your textbook.)*

9. Explain why the nurse used a light to illuminate Sally Begay's neck.

10. When the nurse auscultates Sally Begay's chest for lung sounds, she should focus her assessment on what area of the lung (based on the findings from the admitting Physical & History)?
    a. Right upper lobes
    b. Left lower lobes
    c. Right lower lobes
    d. Left middle lobes

➡️ Now click on **Vital Signs** and observe the nurse as she measures Sally Begay's pulse oximetry and assesses her pain.

11. When the nurse assesses Sally Begay's oxygen saturation, what does she do incorrectly?

12. As a result of the nurse's technique, you would expect Sally Begay's oxygen saturation to be:
    a. falsely high.
    b. falsely low.

13. During the assessment of Sally Begay's chest pain, the nurse asks, "Does it travel to the jaw or shoulders?" The nurse's question is asked to rule out the possibility of chest pain due to:
    a. myocardial infarction.
    b. congestive heart failure.
    c. bronchitis.
    d. pneumonia.

➡️ Exit the patient's room and go to one of the computers that allow you to access the EPR. Open Sally Begay's EPR and review the results of her hematology tests and assessment findings.

14. Note that Sally Begay's hemoglobin and hematocrit values changed from admission to Tuesday morning. The hemoglobin dropped from 13.3 to 12.1 and the hematocrit dropped from 40.1 to 36. This change indicates a risk for:
    a. carbon dioxide retention.
    b. decreased oxygen-carrying capacity of blood.
    c. limited diffusion of oxygen through the alveoli.
    d. increased metabolic rate.

15. While reviewing Sally Begay's assessment findings, identify three assessment measures that you would monitor closely to determine whether there is a change in Sally Begay's oxygenation status.

→ Now return to Sally Begay's room and review her health history.

16. Sally Begay is suffering from a number of medical conditions that are affecting her oxygenation status. To more fully assess her oxygenation needs, you must apply a critical thinking approach. Complete the following diagram by placing the letter of each critical thinking factor under its corresponding category

KNOWLEDGE

(1) _____

(2) _____

(3) _____

(4) _____

EXPERIENCE　　**ASSESSMENT OF OXYGENATION**　　**STANDARDS**

(5) _____

(6) _____

(7) _____

(8) _____

ATTITUDES

(9) _____

(10) _____

Critical Thinking Factors

    a. Accurately measure oxygen saturation with the fingernail site properly prepared.

    b. When assessing Sally Begay's thorax, be thorough in including all appropriate measurements.

    c. Review the relationship congestive heart failure has on the pulmonary circulation.

    d. Review your personal journal for experiences with previous patients with pulmonary problems.

    e. Use laboratory guidelines to determine whether chemistry findings are normal or abnormal.

    f. Review environmental factors that predispose the patient to risk for exposure to the Hantavirus.

    g. Being unfamiliar with Navajo customs, determine the culture's views regarding preventive health practices.

    h. Determine Sally Begay's husband's concerns about his wife's activity tolerance and ability to work on the farm.

    i. When assessing Sally Begay's ability to participate in health management, learn more about what she knows about CHF and bronchitis and how it affects her ability to breath.

    j. Review the clinical signs and symptoms to expect when pulmonary congestion worsens.

17. Being accurate in the selection of nursing diagnoses is important. Review each of the following nursing diagnoses, along with their defining characteristics, and circle the diagnosis that most likely applies to Sally Begay.

Ineffective breathing pattern	**Impaired gas exchange**
Dyspnea	Tachycardia
Orthopnea	Restlessness
Altered chest excursion	Hypoxia
Use of accessory muscles to breathe	Dyspnea
Pursed lip breathing	Hypoxemia
Respiratory rate >24/min	Abnormal rate and depth of breathing

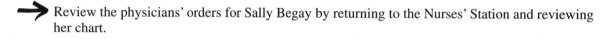 Review the physicians' orders for Sally Begay by returning to the Nurses' Station and reviewing her chart.

18. Sally Begay has had a productive cough since admission. She is able to mobilize secretions. Which of the following interventions would be appropriate for her?
    a. Nasopharyngeal suctioning
    b. Chest physiotherapy
    c. Coughing techniques
    d. Incentive spirometry

19. The physician ordered Sally Begay to be up in a chair and to ambulate. Provide a scientific rationale for why this therapy is appropriate.

20. Why must the nurse be concerned about providing frequent oral care and skin assessment when administering oxygen by nasal cannula?

→ Close the patient's chart and go to the Supervisor's Office. Sign in again on the desktop computer, keeping Sally Begay as your patient but changing your shift to Thursday at 1100. Now go to the mobile computer in the hallway and access Sally Begay's EPR. Click on I&O and review her intake and output data. *(Study Tip: Review Chapter 40 in your textbook.)*

21. After reviewing Sally Begay's I&O data since Sunday, what concerns do you have? What action would you consider taking?

22. Why is it important to confer with Sally Begay's physician about increasing her fluid intake?
    a. An increase in fluids might increase her nausea.
    b. An increase in fluids might worsen her CHF.
    c. An increase in fluids might require continued IV therapy.
    d. An increase in fluids might reduce the thickness of mucus secretions.

Exercise 2 – David Ruskin, Thursday 1100

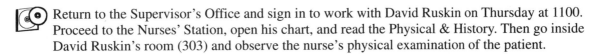 Return to the Supervisor's Office and sign in to work with David Ruskin on Thursday at 1100. Proceed to the Nurses' Station, open his chart, and read the Physical & History. Then go inside David Ruskin's room (303) and observe the nurse's physical examination of the patient.

1. Now that you reviewed the chart data and observed the physical examination, which of the following is the best description of David Ruskin's pulmonary problem?
    a. Decreased chest wall movement
    b. Decreased pulmonary perfusion
    c. Decreased diffusion
    d. Decreased oxygen-carrying capacity

2. As a result of pain affecting David Ruskin's chest wall movement, you would expect which of the following physiologic responses?
    a. Prevents raising of diaphragm and increases anteroposterior diameter of thorax on inspiration
    b. Prevents raising of diaphragm and decreases anteroposterior diameter of the thorax on inspiration
    c. Prevents lowering of diaphragm and increases anteroposterior diameter of the thorax on inspiration
    d. Prevents lowering of diaphragm and reduces anteroposterior diameter of thorax on inspiration

3. Which of the following nursing therapies would be most appropriate to improve David's ability to ventilate more fully?
    a. Increase fluid intake.
    b. Administer oxycodone 30 minutes prior to deep breathing exercises.
    c. Perform chest percussion over the involved right chest wall.
    d. Administer oxygen per nasal cannula with humidification.

4. Aggressive management of David Ruskin's chest pain is designed to prevent:
    a. hypoventilation.
    b. hypoxia.
    c. hyperventilation.
    d. cyanosis.

Exercise 3 – Andrea Wang, Tuesday 1100

 Return to the Supervisor's Office. This time, sign in to work with Andrea Wang for the Tuesday 1100 shift. Go to the Nurses' Station, open her chart (310), and review the Physical & History.

1. A partial transection of the spinal cord at T5 and T6 could lead to what type of nerve paralysis that affects respiration or ventilation?
   a. Paralysis of phrenic nerve
   b. Paralysis of vocal cords
   c. Paralysis of intercostal muscles
   d. Paralysis of peripheral nerves

2. Explain how this type of injury could potentially affect Andrea Wang's ability to receive adequate oxygenation.

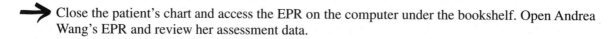 Close the patient's chart and access the EPR on the computer under the bookshelf. Open Andrea Wang's EPR and review her assessment data.

3. Do any findings from Andrea Wang's previous assessments suggest that hypoventilation is a risk for her? If so, explain.

Activity, Mobility, and Skin Integrity

———————————————————————————————

 ✏️ **Reading Assignment:** Activity and Exercise (Chapter 36)
 Mobility and Immobility (Chapter 46)
 Skin Integrity and Wound Care (Chapter 47)
Patients: Ira Bradley, Room 309
 Andrea Wang, Room 310

Objectives

* Discuss the relationship of exercise and physical activity to a patient's health.
* Describe the effects of exercise on body systems.
* Assess factors affecting activity tolerance for patients in the case studies.
* Select appropriate activity interventions for patients in the case studies.
* Identify the effects immobility has on body systems.
* Perform an assessment that identifies potential hazards of immobility for case study patients.
* Assess a patient's risk for skin breakdown.
* Develop a nursing plan of care for a patient with impaired mobility.
* Evaluate nursing interventions designed to improve a patient's activity and mobility.

Activity and regular exercise keep us healthy. When a person develops a health problem that limits normal exercise or creates a temporary or permanent impairment in mobility, almost every body system can be affected. Proper functioning of the musculature and bones, the circulatory system, and other major organ systems such as the skin, heart, and lungs, depend on regular exercise and activity.

Patients within health care settings present a wide variety of activity and mobility limitations: the older adult with degenerative arthritis, the young businessman with ligament damage to the knee, a college student who suffers a paralyzing injury to the spinal cord. As a nurse you must be able to recognize not only how patients' presenting health problems affect their ability to remain active and mobile but also how these problems pose risks for the function of all body systems. Preventive care is a key aspect of supporting a patient's mobility and activity tolerance. Early assessment is especially important as you learn to look for signs of changes reflecting the effects of altered mobility. Application of critical thinking ensures a well-considered plan of care that incorporates nursing interventions to keep patients active and within their limitations and to prevent complications of immobility.

Exercise 1 – Ira Bradley, Tuesday 1100

 Go to the Supervisor's Office (Room 301) and sign in on the desktop computer, selecting Ira Bradley for Tuesday at 1100. Proceed to the Nurses' Station, open his chart (309), and review the Physical & History, scrolling down to read all pages. As you read the Physical & History, begin completing the form in question 1. Then close the chart and access the EPR on the computer under the bookshelf. Continue to complete the form in question 1 as you read Ira Bradley's Admissions Profile and his ADL, assessment, and vital sign summaries.

1. Ira Bradley suffers from a progressive, systemic infection (HIV) that is affecting numerous body systems. In his case the progression of the disease creates risks for the decline of his mobility and activity. Complete the form below to assess physical signs and symptoms indicating risks associated with activity and mobility restriction. If necessary, return to the patient's chart and EPR to complete all areas.

Activity and Mobility Restriction – Risk Assessment

Check all changes that apply to Ira Bradley and describe the changes.

Systemic Effects

___ *Metabolic Changes*
Nutrition/appetite

Infection

___ *Respiratory Changes*
Lung fields

Respiratory pattern

Oxygen-carrying capacity

___ *Cardiovascular Changes*
Heart rate

Activity tolerance

___ *Musculoskeletal Changes*
Strength

Muscle condition

Activity level

(continued)

Activity and Mobility Restriction – Risk Assessment (cont'd)

Check all changes that apply to Ira Bradley and describe the changes.

Systemic Effects

___ *Integumentary Changes*
Skin condition

Mucosa

___ *Gastrointestinal Changes*
Swallowing

___ *Comfort Level Changes*
Sources of pain

2. Ira Bradley's continuous state of exhaustion suggests poor activity tolerance. All of the following factors affect activity tolerance except:
   a. mood.
   b. home environmental setting.
   c. age.
   d. motivation.

3. During ambulation or activities such as bathing and dressing, a patient's intolerance to activity may be assessed by the presence of:
   a. lower heart rate and dyspnea.
   b. fatigue and chest pain.
   c. increased oxygen saturation and bradypnea.
   d. decreased work of breathing and lower heart rate.

4. Ira Bradley has crackles in both lung bases, and on Monday his assessment revealed shallow, labored breathing. If Ira Bradley were to remain inactive, what effects might you see on his pulmonary system?

5. Identify four factors that increase Ira Bradley's risk for a pressure ulcer. *(Study Tip: Review Skill 47-1 in Chapter 47 of your textbook.)*

→   Now go inside Room 309 to visit Ira Bradley. Click on **Health History** and observe the nurse's interview of Ira Bradley.

6. If you were conducting Ira Bradley's health history, what might you explore about his activity tolerance that the nurse did not address?
   a. His ability to do ADL
   b. His ability to acquire rest and to sleep
   c. His feelings about his illness and how they affect his desire to remain active
   d. His perceived level of energy

7. Observation of the health history reveals what potential resource that might improve Ira Bradley's motivation to exercise?

8. After observing Ira Bradley and reviewing his medical history data, what form of exercise do you believe he might benefit from most?
   a. Passive range of motion
   b. Isotonic exercise
   c. Gait training
   d. Isometric exercise

9. Show the physiologic effects of immobility by indicating whether each of the following would increase (mark with ↑) or decrease (mark with ↓).

_____   Wound healing

_____   Heart rate

_____   Urine output

_____   Respiratory rate

_____   Bowel sounds

10. Provide a rationale for why each of the following strategies would benefit Ira Bradley.

   a. Teach breathing skills:

   b. Let the patient move at his own pace:

   c. Know the patient's mobility skills prior to hospitalization:

Exercise 2 – Andrea Wang, Tuesday 1100

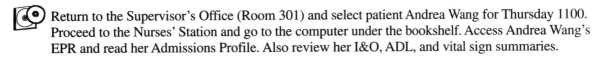 Return to the Supervisor's Office (Room 301) and select patient Andrea Wang for Thursday 1100. Proceed to the Nurses' Station and go to the computer under the bookshelf. Access Andrea Wang's EPR and read her Admissions Profile. Also review her I&O, ADL, and vital sign summaries.

1. The nature of Andrea Wang's mobility alteration is best described as:
   a. postural abnormality.
   b. impaired muscle development.
   c. damage to the central nervous system.
   d. trauma to the musculoskeletal system.

2. Match each of the following changes with the body system(s) affected by immobility. (There may be more than one change in a body system.)

Change	Body System
_____ Negative nitrogen balance	a. Integument
_____ Collapse of alveoli	b. Respiratory
_____ Osteoporosis	c. Musculoskeletal
_____ Thrombus formation	d. Metabolic
_____ Joint contracture	e. Cardiovascular
_____ Reduced strength of cough	
_____ Pressure ulcer	

→ Go to Room 310 to visit Andrea Wang. Click on **Health History** and observe the nurse and patient during interviews in each of the functional health pattern areas. As you review the health history, use the following form to take notes.

Andrea Wang's Health History

Observed behaviors:

Sleep-wake status:

Coping response and resources:

Health perception:

---

3. Andrea Wang reports that she feels exhausted and awakens frequently. What factor related to the management of her immobility might be contributing to her poor sleep quality?

4. Over time Andrea Wang's behavioral response to her spinal cord injury and her coping resources will influence her motivation to stay involved in her therapy. Discuss your view of how to strengthen Andrea Wang's ability to cope with her injury.

5. Application of critical thinking to your assessment of Andrea Wang's health status will ensure a more complete and relevant assessment. Complete the diagram below by writing the letter of each critical thinking factor (listed on next page) under its corresponding category.

KNOWLEDGE

(1) _____

(2) _____

(3) _____

(4) _____

EXPERIENCE

(5) _____

(6) _____

ASSESSMENT

STANDARDS

(7) _____

(8) _____

(9) _____

ATTITUDES

(10) _____

(11) _____

Critical Thinking Factors

   a. Andrea Wang's risk for immobility requires a broad examination of each body system function.

   b. The use of the Braden Scale will determine Andrea Wang's risk for obtaining a pressure ulcer.

   c. Reflect upon the times you have cared for a patient who was restricted to bed because of illness or a treatment.

   d. Physiologic response of the body to spinal shock.

   e. Consider how you felt when forced to remain in a position for too long.

   f. When you assess Andrea Wang, speak with conviction, emphasizing that your questions will help you in better planning her care.

   g. Effect of immobilization on major body systems.

   h. Assessment of range of motion of Andrea Wang's paralyzed extremities should include actual range of movement compared with normal range for each joint.

   i. It will take some effort to position Andrea Wang in a way that allows you to view her skin completely. Take time to be thorough.

   j. Review Andrea Wang's health status prior to the accident.

   k. Know the effect immobility has on a patient's psychosocial well-being.

6. When Andrea Wang is placed in the supine position, there are a number of pressure points over bony prominences where pressure ulcers might develop. On the following figure, identify each circled area where pressure ulcers might develop.

(1) _____

(2) _____

(3) _____

(4) _____

(5) _____

(6) _____

(7) _____

(8) _____

(9) _____

(10) _____

7. Of the areas identified in the figure above, which are least likely to be a problem for Andrea Wang? Provide a rationale for your answer.

→ Return to the Nurses' Station, open Andrea Wang's chart (310) and read the nurses' notes for the last few days.

8. Apply the Braden Scale to what you have learned about Andrea Wang from her health history, EPR, and chart data. *(Study Tip: Refer to Table 47-5 in Chapter 47 of your textbook for help.)*

What score(s) would you assess for Andrea Wang in each of the following areas?

Sensory perception _____

Moisture _____

Activity _____

Mobility _____

Nutrition _____

Friction and shearing _____

9. Now add Andrea Wang's individual scores in question 8. Based on her total Braden scale score, is she at a high or low risk for pressure ulcer development?

   High   Low

10. Review assessment data on Andrea Wang and identify four nursing diagnoses that you believe apply to her neuromuscular injury. Include relevant defining characteristics for each diagnosis.

    Nursing diagnosis   **Defining characteristics**

11. One nursing diagnosis applicable to Andrea Wang's situation is Impaired physical mobility. Review the following nursing plan of care for Andrea Wang, critique it carefully, and identify any inappropriate care recommendations.

Nursing Care Plan

Goal

Patient remains free of complications of immobility.

Outcomes

Patient's range of motion improves.

Patient's skin remains intact, without abnormal reactive hyperemia over bony prominences.

Patient's lung fields remain clear.

Interventions

Change patient's position regularly while awake; position on side, supine, opposite side, with HOB elevated 40 degrees.

Apply egg crate mattress to patient's bed.

Clean and dry skin thoroughly following any episode of incontinence.

Instruct patient on technique for controlled coughing; have patient deep breathe and cough every 1 to 2 hours while awake.

Maintain patient's fluid intake at 1000 ml daily.

Assist patient in performing passive range-of-motion exercises to lower extremities 4 times a day.

Assist patient in performing passive range-of-motion exercises to upper extremities 4 times a day.

Critique of plan:

---

12. Indicate which of the following additional nursing interventions would benefit Andrea Wang in preventing complications of immobility. (Place an **X** next to all interventions that apply.)

_____ Chest physiotherapy

_____ Elastic stockings

_____ Hand rolls

_____ Ankle/foot orthotic device

_____ Monitoring of lab data

13. The first time Andrea Wang is assisted into a wheelchair, it is important to assess for:
    a. Homan's sign.
    b. orthostatic hypotension.
    c. contracture of ankle.
    d. pressure ulcer.

14. When assisting with passive range-of-motion exercises, what does the nurse do to prevent injury to the joint?

15. Match each of the following interventions with the evaluation measure used to determine its effectiveness.

Evaluation Measure	**Intervention**
_____ Apply pressure briefly to skin and observe for blanching.	a. Antiembolism stockings
_____ Measure degrees in full range of a joint's movement.	b. Coughing and turning
_____ Perform dorsiflexion of foot and ask whether patient feels pain in calf.	c. ROM exercises
_____ Auscultate lung fields.	d. Turning and placement on support surface

LESSON 12

Elimination

Reading Assignment: Urinary Elimination (Chapter 44)
Bowel Elimination (Chapter 45)

Patients: Carmen Gonzales, Room 302
Andrea Wang, Room 310

Objectives

- Describe factors that influence normal urination.
- Describe factors that influence normal defecation.
- Identify factors contributing to elimination problems in case study patients.
- Interpret laboratory results of urine testing.
- Discuss implications of diagnostic testing of elimination function.
- Conduct assessment of elimination status of a case study patient.
- Discuss scientific principles applied in urinary elimination nursing interventions.
- Develop a plan of care for a case study patient with elimination alteration.

Normal and regular urinary and bowel elimination are essential for a sense of well-being and healthy body functioning. Alterations in elimination can be warning signs of problems involving other body systems. Because elimination is affected by personal choices and lifestyle habits, patterns of elimination will vary among patients. An important part of nursing care for patients with elimination alterations is recognition of pattern variations, knowledge of normal elimination function, and a sensitivity to patients' needs. Patients may become very embarrassed when they are no longer able to urinate or defecate normally, using toilet facilities.

Many different factors within a health care setting can affect a patient's elimination patterns and habits. Medications, diagnostic treatments, diet, activity, and the pathophysiologic process of disease conditions are just some of the factors that may temporarily or permanently disrupt normal elimination. Timely response to a patient's needs and a caring approach will ensure that you provide your patient with quality care.

Exercise 1 – Carmen Gonzales, Thursday 1100

Begin in the Supervisor's Office (Room 301) by signing in on the desktop computer. Select Carmen Gonzales as your patient for the Thursday 1100 shift. Proceed to the mobile computer in the hallway and open the EPR. Review Carmen Gonzales' Admissions Profile, as well as her assessment data, I&O summary, and urinalysis results.

1. Determine Carmen Gonzales' 24-hour intake and output for Wednesday by providing the following data.

   Intake

      Oral =

      IV fluids =

      Antibiotic fluid =

      24-hour total intake =

   Output

      Urine =

      Stool =

      24-hour total output =

2. Would you evaluate Carmen Gonzales' I&O to be normal or abnormal? Give a rationale.

3. What factor within Carmen Gonzales' medical history explains why it is appropriate for her intake to be less than her output? *(Study Tip: Review Chapter 40 in your textbook.)*
   a. History of coronary artery disease
   b. Hypertension
   c. Treatment for gangrenous left leg
   d. History of congestive heart failure

4. Based on what you read in Carmen Gonzales' Admissions Profile, what factor in her lifestyle might increase her daily urinary output?

5. To conduct a more thorough assessment of Carmen Gonzales' urinary elimination status, review the results of her urinalysis. Would you evaluate the findings from her urinalysis as normal or abnormal?

6. Carmen Gonzales' nurse would have obtained a clean-voided specimen for the urinalysis. What most likely explains the reason that the patient has a trace of bacteria in her urine sample?

→ Close the EPR and go to the Nurses' Station. Find and open Carmen Gonzales' chart (302). Review the Physical & History. (Remember to scroll down to read all pages.) Then close her chart and access the MAR (in the blue notebook on the counter). Review Carmen Gonzales' MAR for the last several days.

7. Which of the following drugs will likely cause increased urination?
   a. Acetaminophen
   b. Furosemide
   c. Cefoxitin
   d. Oxycodone

8. When would be the best time of day to have Carmen Gonzales take a diuretic medication? Give your rationale.

9. Carmen Gonzales' Physical & History reveals that she has which of the following urinary alterations?
   a. Hematuria and dribbling
   b. Dysuria and frequency
   c. Frequency and nocturia
   d. Urgency and oliguria

10. Carmen Gonzales has type 2 diabetes mellitus, a disorder of carbohydrate metabolism resulting in increased blood glucose levels. How does diabetes affect her urination? (*Study Tip: Refer to a pathophysiology textbook in your library.*)

11. A patient's ability to void normally depends on all of the following *except*:
    a. feeling the urge to urinate.
    b. being able to take in fluids.
    c. being able to control the urethral sphincter.
    d. being able to relax during voiding.

12. Match each of the following nursing interventions with its corresponding principle for promoting elimination. (Some principles will be matched with more than one intervention.)

Nursing Intervention	**Principle to promote elimination**
_____ Have patient assume normal position for voiding.	a. Promote bladder emptying
_____ Turn on running water as patient attempts to urinate.	b. Stimulate micturition reflex
_____ Have patient void before a meal, as practiced at home.	c. Maintain elimination habits
_____ Warm the surface of a bedpan.	
_____ Have patient practice pelvic floor exercises.	

→ Close Carmen Gonzales' MAR and review once more her Admissions Profile and I&O data in the EPR. (Remember: You can access this information on the computer under the bookshelf in the Nurses' Station or on the mobile computer outside of Carmen Gonzales' room.)

13. Carmen Gonzales was admitted on Sunday. Her Admissions Profile reports that she had some diarrhea, but her I&O records for the next several days show no episodes of a stool being passed. List three factors that might have taken place during the 24 hours leading to Carmen Gonzales' admission that could have influenced her bowel elimination function.

14. Which of the following is a common cause of constipation?
    a. Regular intake of fruit juices
    b. Intake of a high-fiber diet
    c. Regular exercise
    d. Heavy laxative use

→ Go to Carmen Gonzales' room (302) and observe the nutritional portion of her health history.

15. After reviewing Carmen Gonzales' eating patterns, match each of the following foods with the corresponding fiber content.

Food	**Fiber Content**
_____ Rice	a. Low-fiber
_____ Chicken	b. High-fiber
_____ Broccoli	
_____ Eggs	
_____ Grapefruit	
_____ Beans	

Exercise 2 – Andrea Wang, Thursday 1100

 Return to the Supervisor's office (Room 301) to sign in for a new patient. This time, select Andrea Wang for Thursday at 1100. Proceed to the Nurses' Station and open Andrea Wang's chart (310). Review her Physical & History and the physician's orders.

1. A review of Andrea Wang's Physical & History shows she has suffered a partial transection of the thoracic spinal cord and temporary spinal shock. Injury to the spinal cord disrupts voluntary impulses traveling from the brain to the spinal cord. Spinal shock causes loss of autonomic innervation. As a result, she is demonstrating which of the following physical alterations? (Place an **X** next to all that apply.)

   _____ Reduced rectal sphincter tone

   _____ Reduced sense of bladder fullness

   _____ Reduced urethral sphincter tone

   _____ Reduced peristalsis

2. Because Andrea Wang is unable to control micturition, the appropriate therapy at this time is:
   a. strengthening pelvic floor muscles.
   b. creating a flexible toileting schedule.
   c. inserting an indwelling urinary catheter.
   d. Using Credé's method.

3. The physicians' orders show that the Foley catheter was discontinued on Sunday but then the catheter was ordered to be reinserted on Monday. If Andrea Wang has a spinal cord injury, why was the catheter discontinued?

4. Note that the physician had recommended on Sunday to replace the indwelling Foley catheter with bladder scanning and use of a straight catheter. What likely involves bladder scanning?

5. Which of the following was the likely indication for the order to use a straight catheter for Andrea Wang?
   a. Obstruction to urine outflow
   b. Measurement of urine output
   c. Treatment of skin ulcer or wound irritated by urine
   d. Routine intermittent drainage of the bladder

6. Describe the rationale for use of a straight catheter in the long term management of patients with spinal cord damage.

7. The insertion of a Foley catheter creates a potential risk for infection. Match each of the following nursing actions with its corresponding scientific rationale.

Nursing Action

_____ Maintain retraction of labial tissues throughout procedure for catheter insertion.

_____ Cleanse urethral meatus from center of meatus outward or from meatus toward anus.

_____ Hold catheter securely with sterile glove until balloon is inflated.

_____ Attach catheter securely to tubing of drainage bag.

_____ Position drainage bag on bed frame below level of bladder with tubing looped on mattress.

Scientific Rationale

a. Prevents accidental expulsion from bladder, requiring reinsertion

b. Establishes closed system for urine drainage

c. Prevents contamination of meatus during cleansing

d. Removes microorganisms from area of least contamination to area of most contamination

e. Prevents buildup of urine in bladder and pooling of urine in drainage tubing

➤ Close Andrea Wang's chart and access her EPR on the computer below the bookshelf. Review her I&O data and Admissions Profile.

8. Andrea Wang is able to maintain a normal fluid intake, but the volume of urine in the drainage collection bag is consistently low. What might be the problem, and what could you do to correct it?

9. Compute Andrea Wang's 24-hour I&O totals for Wednesday.

Intake

       Oral =

       IV fluids =

Output

       Urine =

       Stool =

       Other =

Net for 24 hours =

➤ Close the EPR and proceed to Room 310 to visit Andrea Wang. Review her health history, focusing primarily on elimination, nutrition, health perception, and coping and stress.

10. Andrea Wang is obviously embarrassed by the incontinence she has experienced. She has likely had incontinent stool and she might have had overflow incontinence during the time the Foley was removed and then reinserted. Identify three nursing measures you would institute to minimize the embarrassment from incontinence. Give a rationale for each measure.

Nursing Measure   **Rationale**

11. Considering Andrea Wang's situation, match each of the following factors with its corresponding effect on bowel elimination.

Factor	**Effect on Bowel Elimination**
_____ Immobilization from paralysis	a. Increased peristalsis
_____ Anger and fear from loss of ability to walk	b. Decreased peristalsis
_____ Increased fluid intake	
_____ Decreased food intake	

→ Return to the Nurses' Station and open the MAR (in the blue notebook on the counter). Review Andrea Wang's current medications.

12. For what purpose is docusate sodium prescribed?

13. When a patient is at risk for bowel and urinary incontinence, the primary nursing care problem that must be prevented is:
a. fluid and electrolyte imbalance
b. flatulence
c. infection
d. impaired skin integrity

14. If, during your care of Andrea Wang, you were to notice that her stool was black in color, what should you do? Why?

LESSON _____ **13** _____

Loss and Grief and Nursing Interventions to Support Coping

_____

Reading Assignment: Responding to Loss, Death, and Grieving (Chapter 29)
Stress and Adaptation (Chapter 30)

Patients: Andrea Wang, Room 310
David Ruskin, Room 303
Ira Bradley, Room 309

Objectives

- Describe loss and the grief responses that patients experience.
- Distinguish among the types of losses.
- Explain the relationship between loss and stress.
- Describe coping mechanisms used by patients in the case studies.
- Assess patients' responses to grief.
- Develop a nursing plan of care for a patient experiencing grief.
- Define ways to evaluate a patient's success in coping with loss.

When a patient experiences a loss, the psychologic impact can be devastating. However a loss for one person (e.g., the death of a pet, moving away from a friend) may not be a loss for another person; the experience is unique. Loss comes in many forms based on the values and priorities of each person's sphere of influence, including family, friends, work associates, society, and cultural environment. When a loss occurs, a person responds emotionally and behaviorally through the grief process. Grief is manifested in a variety of ways that are individual and based on personal experiences, values, cultural expectations, and spiritual beliefs. Over time the grief process allows a person to gradually accept and adapt to loss in order to move on in life. The concepts of stress and adaptation apply to patients who experience loss because the response to loss can cause serious physical and psychologic stress. Therefore coping resources become important when a person struggles to deal with loss.

As a nurse you will experience caring for patients and families who have had all types of losses. The individual patient's coping resources and the severity or type of loss will influence the grief response and the patient's ability to adapt. Your challenge will be to accept the loss as something that is unique and meaningful to the patient and to adapt nursing interventions that will enable the patient to successfully grieve and cope with the loss.

Exercise 1 – Andrea Wang, Thursday 1100

 Begin in the Supervisor's Office (Room 301) by signing in on the desktop computer and selecting Andrea Wang as your patient for Thursday at 1100. Proceed to the Nurses' Station and open her chart (310). First read the Physical & History, scrolling down to read all pages. Then read the nurses' notes.

1. Now that you have reviewed Andrea Wang's chart, what type of loss describes her spinal cord injury?
   a. Maturational
   b. Situational
   c. Actual
   d. Perceived

2. As a result of her paralysis, Andrea Wang is threatened with experiencing other losses. Name three of these potential losses.

3. Andrea Wang's accident occurred about a week ago. Can you predict what stage of grieving she might be experiencing now? Explain why or why not.

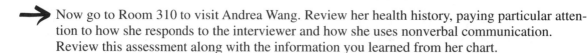 Now go to Room 310 to visit Andrea Wang. Review her health history, paying particular attention to how she responds to the interviewer and how she uses nonverbal communication. Review this assessment along with the information you learned from her chart.

4. Identify three nonverbal responses Andrea Wang conveyed during the health history interview.

5. There are many psychologic indicators of stress. Refer to Box 30-4 in your textbook. List three psychologic indicators revealed in your assessment of Andrea Wang so far.

6. As you listened to Andrea Wang's responses throughout the health history, what did she express in regards to hope? Describe examples in detail.

Study Tip: Review a reference on spinal cord transection: the physiology, clinical signs and symptoms, and prognosis.

7. Andrea Wang is obviously experiencing a very significant loss. To more fully assess her grief response, you must apply a critical thinking approach. Complete the diagram below by writing the letter of each critical thinking factor under its corresponding category.

KNOWLEDGE

(1) _____

(2) _____

(3) _____

EXPERIENCE   **ASSESSMENT OF**   **STANDARDS**
             GRIEF RESPONSE

(4) _____   (6) _____

(5) _____   (7) _____

ATTITUDES

(8) _____

(9) _____

Critical Thinking Factors
   a. Respect Andrea Wang's right to determine how to involve Eric and her parents in an assessment of her needs.
   b. Before assessing Andrea Wang's feelings about sexuality, recognize that you may need more information from a clinical expert on the subject.
   c. Apply what you have learned as a young adult in terms of the importance of relationships with friends.
   d. Know the effects of spinal shock and the responses to expect once it is resolved.
   e. To learn the full extent of how paralysis might affect Andrea Wang, have her describe what she typically did during a school day and a work day.
   f. Andrea Wang has shown embarrassment over her incontinence; therefore approach the assessment by maintaining her dignity and self-esteem.
   g. Review the caring processes in Swanson's theory of caring.
   h. If you have cared for a patient who has lost function of a body part, apply what you learned when you assess Andrea Wang.
   i. Apply what you know about the stages of grief Andrea Wang is experiencing as you phrase your assessment questions.

8. Which of the following questions or statements would be appropriate to assess Andrea Wang's parents' ability to provide meaningful support in helping their daughter face the problems posed by her paralysis?
   a. "Andrea tells us that you do not work things out together. Can you tell me more?"
   b. "Have you thought about how you can help once Andrea returns home?"
   c. "Now is a very difficult time for Andrea . You seem reluctant to visit her in her room."
   d. "Tell me what concerns you have about Andrea's injury and how it will affect her."

9. List three questions you might use to assess the ability of Andrea Wang's boyfriend Eric to provide support for her. *(Study Tip: Refer to Table 29-2 in your textbook.)*

 10. Which of the following indicators requires more exploration during the health history to assess the effect Andrea Wang's injury has had on her level of stress? *(Study Tip: Refer to your textbook for explanations of these indicators.)*
   a. Emotional/behavioral indicator
   b. Intellectual indicator
   c. Lifestyle indicator
   d. Spiritual indicator

→ The health care team can be a valuable asset in determining the type of needs Andrea Wang has and in forming a comprehensive plan of care. Go to Room 308 to listen to each health team member's report. Then proceed to the Nurses' Station, open Andrea Wang's chart (310), and click on **Health Team** to review their written reports.

11. Review your assessment findings to develop a nursing diagnosis for Andrea Wang. Two possible nursing diagnoses are Ineffective individual coping and Hopelessness. Review the following lists of defining characteristics for these two diagnoses. Place an **X** next to all those that apply to Andrea Wang.

Ineffective individual coping	**Hopelessness**
_____ Lack of goal-directed behavior/ resolution of problem	_____ Passivity; decreased verbalization
_____ Sleep disturbance	_____ Decreased affect
_____ Decreased use of social support	_____ Verbal cues (e.g., sighing; saying, "I feel so helpless.")
_____ Use of coping mechanisms that impede adaptive behavior	_____ Closing eyes
_____ Fatigue	_____ Decreased appetite
_____ Inadequate problem solving	_____ Decreased response to stimuli
_____ Verbalization of inability to cope	_____ Increased/decreased sleep
_____ Inability to meet basic needs	_____ Lack of initiative
_____ Destructive behavior towards self and others	_____ Lack of involvement in care
_____ Inability to meet role expectations	_____ Shrugging in response to speaker
_____ Risk taking	

Based on your choices, which nursing diagnosis do you think best applies to Andrea Wang at this time?

12. Andrea Wang is obviously a complicated case. Review what you have learned from the Physical & History, nurses' notes, information from the health team, and the health history. Based on this, list four additional nursing diagnoses you believe apply to her case.

 13. Using Ineffective individual coping as your nursing diagnosis, develop a plan of care for Andrea Wang. *(Study Tip: Refer to possible planning and implementation guidelines in Chapters 29 and 30 in your textbook.)*

Nursing Diagnosis: Ineffective individual coping

Goals   **Expected Outcomes**

Interventions   **Rationale**

Evaluation

14. Paralysis is a devastating injury. Reflect for a moment as to how such an injury might affect *your* life. Identify four changes that paralysis would create in your own life and discuss what you think you would require to cope with each of those changes.

Exercise 2 – David Ruskin, Thursday 1100

 Return to the Supervisor's Office (Room 301) and select David Ruskin as your patient for Thursday at 1100. Go to the mobile computer in the hallway, access his EPR, and review his Admissions Profile. Then proceed to David Ruskin's room (303) and review his health history.

1. David Ruskin's injury was acute and probably caused immediate, acute pain. Which of the following physiologic responses to the stress of the injury most likely occurred?
   a. Increased heart rate
   b. Decreased gluconeogenesis
   c. Decreased mental acuity
   d. Decreased blood pressure

2. David Ruskin's Admissions Profile summarizes a brief history collected at the time of his admission to the hospital. Match each of the following assessment findings with its corresponding type of coping factor.

Assessment Finding	**Type of Coping Factor**
_____ Talks things over with his wife	a. Intellectual factor
_____ Requests information about injury	b. Lifestyle factor
_____ Uncertain how ADL will be affected	c. Family factor
_____ Knows his injury will affect triathlon training	

3. What stage of grieving, based upon Rando's theory of grief do you suspect David Ruskin is experiencing?
   a. Avoidance
   b. Accommodation
   c. Developing awareness
   d. Anger

4. Compare David Ruskin's loss with that of Andrea Wang's in Exercise 1. Do you believe David Ruskin will experience grief over his injury? Explain.

Exercise 3 – Ira Bradley, Thursday 1100

 Go to the Supervisor's Office (Room 301) to sign in again on the desktop computer. This time, select Ira Bradley as your patient for the Thursday 1100 shift. Proceed to the Nurses' Station, open his chart, and read the Physical & History. Then go to Room 309 to visit Ira Bradley. Observe the nurse and the patient during the health history interview.

1. Complete the following data sheet, describing what you learned about Ira Bradley in each of these areas of assessment.

---

a. Ira Bradley's type of loss is:

b. Phase of grief (Kübler-Ross):

Assessment of Factors Influencing Grieving

c. Social support system:

d. Spiritual beliefs:

e. Loss of personal life goals:

f. Family's grief:

---

2. If you had the opportunity to interview Ira Bradley's wife directly, list four questions you might ask that pertain to how her husband's illness is affecting *her*.

3. Ira Bradley presents a number of physical problems because of his illness. Match each of the following comfort measures with nursing care problem(s) it applies to. (Comfort measures may apply to more than one problem.)

Nursing Care Problem	Comfort measures
_____ Fatigue	a. Offer preferred liquids and ice chips.
_____ Pain	b. Provide smaller, more frequent portions of food.
_____ Hydration	c. Provide frequent mouth care.
_____ Appetite	d. Offer analgesic mouthwash.
	e. Pace ordered nursing activities throughout the day.
	f. Control extraneous noise within room environment.
	g. Avoid serving meals when patient's mouth pain is severe.

4. Because Ira Bradley is experiencing depression in his response to grieving, it is most appropriate for you as the nurse to:
   a. offer to stay with him without discussing reasons for his behavior.
   b. listen attentively and provide empathy.
   c. assist in discussing future plans.
   d. focus on providing basic care.

5. When a patient is moving towards acceptance of loss, nursing interventions focus on:
   a. providing anticipatory guidance in helping the patient deal with anger.
   b. providing information for decision making.
   c. avoiding emotional support that reinforces denial.
   d. assisting in verbalizing and discussing future plans.

LESSON 14

Self-Concept

Reading Assignment: Self-Concept (Chapter 26)

Patients: Andrea Wang, Room 310
Ira Bradley, Room 309

Objectives

- Identify components of self-concept.
- Differentiate among self-concept, body image, and self-esteem.
- Identify stressors affecting the self-concept of patients in the case studies.
- Describe ways a nurse can enhance a patient's self-concept.
- Apply critical thinking in developing a plan of care for a patient who has an altered self-concept.

What we think and feel about ourselves affects how we care for ourselves physically and emotionally—and the way we care for others. The knowledge we have gathered about ourselves from our unconscious and conscious thoughts, experiences with others, attitudes, values, and perceptions comprises our self-concept. As a nurse it is important for you to know that a person's self-concept influences his or her perception of health. Illness, loss, and unplanned diagnostic procedures are just a few events that can affect a person's self-concept. For example, chronic illness may change a patient's role in the family, thereby affecting the individual's self-worth and the way in which the family offers support and guidance. When you care for patients, learn whether they have a healthy self-concept, how their health problems influences their self-concept, and the best nursing approaches to maintain or strengthen their self-concept.

Exercise 1 – Andrea Wang, Tuesday 1100

Go to the Supervisor's Office (Room 301) and sign in to work with Andrea Wang as your patient for Tuesday at 1100. Then go to Room 307 to listen to the change-of-shift report on your patient. After listening to report, proceed to the Nurses' Station and access Andrea Wang's EPR on the computer under the bookshelf. Read the Admissions Profile.

137

1. Andrea Wang has suffered a spinal cord injury causing paralysis below the level of the fifth and sixth thoracic vertebra. As you review information from the change-of-shift report and Admissions Profile, what stressors can you identify in the following four categories that have potentially influenced the patient's self-concept?

   a. Body image:

   b. Role:

   c. Self-esteem:

   d. Identity:

➤ Now go to Room 310 and observe Andrea Wang's health history interview. Listen not only to what Andrea Wang says but also to how she conveys her feelings to the nurse.

2. Based on what you learn from the health history, make notes below to identify how components of Andrea Wang's self-concept are influenced by her injury and response to paralysis.

Identity:

Body image:

Self-esteem:

Role performance:

---

3. The best description of self-concept is:
   a. a person's self appraisal of relationships with other individuals.
   b. the roles an individual assumes in life.
   c. a combination of variables that provides a sense of wholeness and consistency for a person.
   d. a person's perception of his or her body.

4. In the case of Andrea Wang, the potential influence of her injury at the present time is most likely to be:
   a. role overload.
   b. role conflict.
   c. role ambiguity.
   d. role strain.

5. Which of the following behaviors did you observe Andrea Wang display, suggesting that she might be experiencing an altered self-concept?
   a. Avoidance of eye contact
   b. Unkempt appearance
   c. Anger
   d. Passive attitude

6. Identify three approaches by which you as a nurse could minimize the stress Andrea Wang is feeling about her self-concept.

   a.

   b.

   c.

7. On the basis of your assessment of Andrea Wang so far, which of the following best describes her normal coping behavior when a problem develops?
   a. She relies on spiritual support to deal with problems.
   b. She works out any difficulties by sharing them with family members.
   c. She avoids asking questions or seeking information.
   d. She prefers to have knowledge made available that she can consider and think through.

8. As you consider developing a plan of care for Andrea Wang, demonstrate how you would apply critical thinking by writing the letter of each critical thinking factor under its corresponding correct category.

KNOWLEDGE

(1) _____

(2) _____

EXPERIENCE   **PLANNING**   **STANDARDS**

(3) _____   (4) _____

ATTITUDES

(5) _____

(6) _____

Critical Thinking Factors

a. Respect Andrea Wang's dignity and privacy when you plan interactions with her and her family.
b. Apply principles of family nursing.
c. In selecting interventions, use what you have learned from patients who have had major surgery or injury.
d. Be informed as to the services a social worker might be able to provide Andrea Wang.
e. After determining who is Andrea Wang's closest ally and support (e.g., Eric or a parent) find approaches to involve this person in your nursing care.
f. Adjustment to paralysis takes time; set goals that are realistic and achievable for the patient.

→ Exit the patient's room and return to the Supervisor's Office (Room 301). Reselect Andrea Wang as your patient, but change your shift to Thursday at 0700. Proceed to Room 308 to listen to the health team meeting. After listening to each member's report, go to the Nurses' Station and open Andrea Wang's chart (310). Click on **Health Team** and read the written reports.

9. The case manager has identified a nursing diagnosis of Ineffective individual coping for Andrea Wang. Based upon your assessment so far, match each of the following defining characteristics for that diagnosis with the patient's corresponding behaviors.

Defining Characteristic	**Patient Behavior**
_____ Verbalization of inability to cope	a. Sarcastically responds to nurse's suggestion to talk about bowel function.
_____ Inability to meet role expectations	b. Says, "I can feed myself now and move my arms a bit."
_____ Inability to meet basic needs	c. Says, "I don't know what is going to happen to me."
_____ Change in usual communication pattern	d. Has concern that she will get behind in school.
_____ Expression of anxiety, depression, impatience	e. Says, "Deep down, I feel exhausted, and helpless."

10. Based on the health team members' recommendations and your own assessment of Andrea Wang's situation, develop a plan of care for the nursing diagnosis of Ineffective individual coping.

Nursing Diagnosis: Ineffective individual coping

Goals   **Expected Outcomes**

Interventions   **Rationale**

Evaluation

Exercise 2 – Ira Bradley, Thursday 1100

Return to the Supervisor's Office (Room 301) and sign in to work with Ira Bradley on Thursday at 1100. Then go to one of the computers that allow you to access the EPR. Open the EPR and review Ira Bradley's Admissions Profile.

1. Match each finding from Ira Bradley's Admissions Profile with the self-concept area affected by that finding. (Each finding may affect more than one self-concept area.)

Finding	Self-Concept Area
_____ Receives treatment for depression	a. Body image
_____ Needs assistance with ADL	b. Role
_____ Senses change in masculinity	c. Identity
_____ Has late-stage HIV	d. Self-esteem
_____ Is fearful of a painful death	

→ Now go inside Room 309 to visit Ira Bradley and his wife. Review his health history findings.

2. While you are observing the health history interview, which of the following behaviors do you notice that suggest Ira Bradley has an altered self-concept? (Place an **X** next to all behaviors that apply.)

_____ Shows anger

_____ Has a passive attitude

_____ Avoids eye contact

_____ Puts himself down

_____ Has an unkempt appearance

3. As you observe Ira Bradley's wife, what type of support or coping does she provide? Can she be a resource in a plan of care? Write a short answer and give your rationale.

4. If you were to conduct the assessment of Ira Bradley, explain how you might apply each of the following critical thinking attitudes.

a. Confidence:

b. Risk taking:

→ Exit the patient's room and go to Room 308 to listen to the health team meeting on Ira Bradley. After you listen to the reports, go to the Nurses' Station and open his chart. Click on **Health Team** and review the written report submitted by each health team member.

5. What additional specific self-concept stressors were identified by members of the health team?

Body image stressors:

Role stressors:

Self-esteem stressors:

Identity stressors:

6. For a man Ira Bradley's age, which of the following developmental factors is more likely to influence his self-concept?
   a. At this time in his life, self-concept and body image are significantly affected by societal approval and acceptance.
   b. This is a normal time for reflection in which Ira Bradley will review his past successes and disappointments in life.
   c. At this stage of his life, it is normal to reassess life experiences and redefine his self-identity in life roles.
   d. At this time, there is a focus on development of identity.

7. Based on the recommendations of the health team, how would you approach patient teaching for Ira Bradley and his family? List three teaching approaches.

Answers

Lesson 1 – Critical Thinking and Nursing Judgment

Exercise 1

1. Your data form should look something like this:
   Diagnosis(es): Infected leg, gangrene, osteomyelitis, diabetes, left-sided heart failure
   Vital Signs: BP 145/80   RR 18–20   HR 20–25 O_2 Sat 90–95
   Recent Medications: Diuretic yesterday; oxycodone yesterday
   Physical Findings: Lungs congested
   Lab Results: Blood glucose 150

2. The correct answers are as follows: b, c, a.

3. The correct answer is choice a. The report of vital sign values provides precise measures to be used in comparing the patient's physical status over time.

4. The correct answer is choice c. The entry in the chart recommending diabetes education is a clinical decision. The nurse completing the Admissions Profile reviewed Carmen Gonzales' clinical problem and recommended an approach believed to be the best one to solve the patient's recurrent leg infection. An educational approach might minimize the severity of the problem (help achieve diabetic control with fewer complications). It is unlikely that it will resolve the problem completely.

5. There are many aspects of knowledge to consider. You need to know more about the patient's culture and how that might influence her interest in education or desire to learn about diabetes management. A knowledge of family nursing, specifically the role families play in a patient's health, is an excellent knowledge base to help you in assessing whether education will be successful for this patient. In addition, a knowledge of patient education principles, including motivation to learn, is critical.

145

6. There are several questions you might ask to assess Carmen Gonzales' pain more thoroughly. These are examples:
   a. Clear—Ask what type of pain the patient experiences.
   b. Relevant—As you assess pain, know that for the patient it is very relevant and real. Ask how the pain affects activities of daily living, mobility, sleep, etc.
   c. Precise—The best way to measure pain is to rate the intensity, on a scale of 0 to 10. *(Study tip: Review Chapter 42 in Fundamentals of Nursing.)*
   d. Consistent—To be consistent over time, use the same measures. Measure intensity using the same pain scale each time so that you can compare findings.

7. Perseverance involves exploring for more information. When Carmen Gonzales made the comment, "I don't know if I'll ever be able to walk again," the nurse should have inquired more as to why she holds such a fear. Instead the fear was ignored.

8. Carmen Gonzales had told the nurse that she did not feel comfortable discussing sexuality. Nonetheless, the nurse explored her health maintenance behaviors and asked her whether her illness affected her relationship with her husband. This information is vital for understanding the patients' health habits and the effect of her illness on her relationship with her husband. Such information has implications for health education and psychosocial support interventions.

9. Part of critical thinking is to analyze data and then interpret. Carmen Gonzales has revealed important information. She has a real fear of not being able to walk again because of her leg; she is fatigued, in pain, and knows her infection continues to recur. Her illness has affected her ability to perform normal activities at home, even though her husband helps. When stressed by illness, she is less able to care for herself or her husband. When analyzing this information, it holds even greater meaning when you learn that Carmen Gonzales' family is most important to her. She is likely afraid of how this illness will affect her ability to retain the role she plays in the family. She faces serious potential losses unless her disease can be better controlled and the infection cleared.

10. Applying critical thinking to Carmen Gonzales' case requires you to consider knowledge and experience and to use attitudes and standards that allow you to collect a strong, comprehensive data base. Answers to the diagram are as follows:
    (1) d—Knowledge of diet components helps to assess diet deficiencies.
    (2) f—Know how health beliefs influence desire to learn.
    (3) h—Cultural influences affect how people choose to learn and accept help.
    (4) b—Reflection allows you to learn from experience.
    (5) c—American Diabetes Association sets education standards.
    (6) g—Be sure assessment is in-depth and thorough.
    (7) a—Use creativity in your assessment approach.
    (8) e—Responsibility: confer with others when you know you need more data.

11. Question a is close-ended and does not encourage elaboration or detailed description. Questions b and c are open-ended; they encourage the patient to describe her eating patterns and her food preferences.

12. There are several interpretations you can make that would require further inquiry: (a) Carmen Gonzales feels hopeless because of her recurrent leg infections and the threat they pose to her ability to walk and remain active. (b) The patient has not managed her diabetes very well through her diet. (c) Carmen Gonzales has many physical reasons for feeling fatigued (heart disease, infection, poor diabetes control, poor sleep) in addition to her overriding sense of hopelessness.

13. As the nurse, you should probe more to assess specifically why she feels she will be unable to walk, what she knows about her diabetes and its relationship to her health problems (specifically her leg infection), and whether she understands how diet management can improve diabetic control.

14. The entry does meet the definition for *subjective data*. The description of the patient's pain comes from Carmen Gonzales. Her pain rating is a bit tricky. Remember, the pain intensity of 8 is a self-report measure and thus subjective, even though you as the nurse can use this measure to compare with other self-reports in the future.

Exercise 2

1. In reviewing Andrea Wang's assessment, the nurse uses different strategies to gather information. The correct order of answers is as follows: d, c, b, a. Example a is an open-ended question that encourages the patient to describe her feelings and concerns. Example d, in contrast, is a closed-ended question that could be answered simply with a yes or no response. Example b followed example a in the interview and is an attempt to focus on Andrea Wang's disbelief over her accident. Example c is the nurse's attempt to offer information about her bowel and bladder problems.

2. It is important in critical thinking to continuously listen and analyze what your patient is saying to you so that you can interpret meaning. In other words, as the patient reveals more information, she is telling a story about her health problems and concerns.

    In the responses listed, Andrea Wang is beginning to reveal information that you can cluster and interpret in a pattern. Cues a, d, e, and f reveal grief over loss. Cue g shows anger. Cues b and c reflect a feeling of hopelessness. Andrea Wang is experiencing grief over the loss of movement in her lower extremities. She does not know whether the paralysis is permanent. Her disbelief, hope, uncertainty, and thoughts for the future are all part of the grief reaction. Anger is present in her response to the nurse's offering to explore the changes that occur with bowel and bladder function. Anger can be a part of grief as well. Hopelessness is a situation in which a person does not feel she has alternatives. Her statements in b and c are more reflective of someone who feels she cannot mobilize energy to take action.

3. Answers to the diagram are as follows: (1) b, (2) d, (3) i, (4) f, (5) h, (6) a, (7) c, (8) g, and (9) e. When applying critical thinking to assessing Andrea's Wang's grief, refer to knowledge of the grief response, the physiology and long-term implications of spinal cord injuries, and knowledge pertaining to the developmental needs of a young adult. This information will allow you to understand the extent of her injury, the behaviors to expect from grieving and potential interventions, and the degree to which the loss will influence the patient's relationship with Eric and her family. When you think critically in this case, apply experience from any personal loss as well as notes you kept after caring for a patient with a similarly meaningful loss. Apply the ethical standard of acquiring Andrea's consent before you interview Eric about their relationship. The intellectual standards of deep and complete ensures that your assessment of Andrea's feelings about the accident is as thorough as possible. You apply the attitude of creativity when conducting a family conference. Finally, using the attitude of discipline ensures you have a thorough sleep history.

4. In an environmental history, you want to learn what you can about Andrea Wang's home environment. What type of residence does she live in? Are there stairs to climb? Is the home arranged in a way that permits wheelchair access from room to room? This information will help to anticipate the patient's needs and how the family might be able to help. Once she does go to rehab, this assessment will be detailed by the physical therapist.

Lesson 2 – Applying the Nursing Process

Exercise 1

1. Your data form should look something like this:
   Patient's Name: *David Ruskin*
   Diagnosis: *Bike accident, open reduction internal fixation (ORIF) of right humerus*
   Vital Signs: Temp *99° F* BP *no data* HR *no data* RR *no data* O$_2$ sat *90% to 92% room air*
   Patient Data (Signs and Symptoms):
      Slept
      Pain in left arm and side
      Breathes regularly, hurts some to breathe
      Lungs clear
      IV left hand
      States he has lot of aches and pains
      Negative Homan's sign, pulses palpable, legs warm
      Abrasions present, no infection
   Mental Status: *Alert and oriented to person and place*

2. The correct order of answers is O, S, S, O, O.

3. Assessment begins by organizing your data into logical patterns. One way to do this is by body systems:
   Circulation
   Negative Homan's sign
   Palpable pulses
   Extremities warm

   Respiration
   Lungs clear
   Breathing regular
   Hurts some to breathe

   Comfort
   Pain in left arm and side
   States he has lot of aches and pains
   Hurts some to breathe

   Skin
   IV in left hand
   Abrasions present, no infection

4. There are many questions that you might consider asking, given the data from David Ruskin's report. Here are a few examples:

Data	Questions to Ask
Respiration	
Lungs clear	Does the pain limit your ability to breathe deeply?
Breathing regular	Are you able to cough without pain?
Hurts some to breathe	Are both sides of the chest affected, or only one side?
	Do you have less pain by lying on the side that hurts?

Comfort

Pain in left arm and side	How severe is your pain on a scale of 0 to 10, with 0 being no pain and 10 being the worst pain you have ever felt?
States he has a lot of aches and pains	
Hurts some to breathe	

How severe is your pain on a scale of 0 to 10, with 0 being no pain and 10 being the worst pain you have ever felt?
Where exactly is the pain located?
Does the pain limit your activities (e.g., turning, bathing)?
Does anything relieve the pain?

Skin

IV in left hand
Abrasions, no infection

What is condition of IV site?
Where are abrasions located?
Are the abrasions a source of discomfort?
What is the appearance of the abrasions?

5. David Ruskin may have the problems of pain, difficulty breathing, and potential infection at either the IV site or site of abrasions.

6. **Pain:** The Admissions Profile reveals that David Ruskin complains of acute pain. The vital signs flow sheet shows that from Monday to Tuesday the patient reported pain on a scale from 7 down to 5. He has constant aching. The Admissions Profile also shows that he has right rib cage pain.
   Difficulty breathing: David Ruskin's Admissions Profile reveals that respirations were guarded at the time of admission, with right rib cage pain. In addition, although his chest expansion was within defined limits the first 2 days, respirations are shallow on Tuesday.
   Potential infection: There is no information about the IV site. However the Admissions Profile reveals there is also a laceration of the scalp. Abrasions are affecting the calf and flank, although the EPR does not identify right or left side.

7. The correct answer is choice b. The pain rating scale (0 to 10) provides the most objective measure of pain for comparison in the future.

8. The correct order of answers is as follows: b, a, a, b, b, b

9. All elements of critical thinking apply when you assess and diagnose your patients. In this example, using critical thinking ensures a thorough assessment and ultimate selection of a diagnosis for David Ruskin's situation. Answers to the diagram are as follows:
   (1) c—Pathophysiology
   (2) e—Wound healing process
   (3) h—Pain characteristics
   (4) d—Experience with similar patients
   (5) a—Precise
   (6) f—Relevance
   (7) b—Discipline
   (8) g—Confidence

10. The correct answer is choice c. This is the etiology within the domain of nursing practice.

11. The correct answer is choice c. The diagnosis as stated commits an error because the etiology is a medical diagnosis. The correct nursing diagnosis would address the patient's response to the surgical procedure.

12. An actual health problem is one that is perceived or experienced by the patient at the time of the nurse's assessment. Pain is an actual problem David Ruskin is currently experiencing. An at-risk health problem is one that the nurse determines a patient is vulnerable to develop.

13. Risk for infection.

14. Among the three nursing diagnoses, Pain is the priority because it currently limits David Ruskin's mobility and it is the etiology for the diagnosis of Ineffective breathing pattern. Control or resolution of the pain would help the patient recover quickly since he is young, healthy, has no chronic disease, and suffered no internal injuries from his accident. The diagnosis of Risk for infection will cause you to take preventive measures in David Ruskin's care—including regular care of the IV site until it is discontinued, keeping all wounds clean (surgical wounds as well as traumatic wounds to the scalp and leg), and maintaining adequate nutritional intake.

15. An example of a goal statement is: Patient will achieve acceptable relief in pain by discharge.

16. The correct answer is choice d. Choices a and b might apply to David Ruskin, but they are not written in measurable terms. Choice c does not ensure that pain is relieved, only that fewer analgesics might be used. Choice d is realistic and measurable, and it could be mutually set with the patient.

17. An example of an appropriate goal: Patient will achieve full lung expansion by discharge. Outcomes might include the following:
    - Chest excursion will increase from 3 to >4 cm within 24 hours. *(Study Tip: Review Chapter 16.)*
    - Respiratory pattern will return to normal within 24 hours.

18. Two physician interventions would include analgesics and elevation of the arm through the use of a sling. (Elevation reduces swelling, which aggravates pain in the tissues.)

19. The correct order of answers is P, N, N, N, P.

20. You can evaluate David Ruskin's pain by administering a pain scale, measuring chest excursion, assessing his respiratory pattern for depth, and observing movement (turning, repositioning of arm).

21. a. Unchanged (full)
    b. Yes
    c. No
    d. Yes

22. The correct answer is choice b. The evaluation shows David Ruskin is still having painful movement. Your best course of action, after having evaluated the patient's response to care, is to continue the current plan, which includes analgesics and placement of his right arm in a sling. In addition, new interventions aimed at adapting the way he repositions and moves, use of splinting, and perhaps administering analgesics prior to ambulation, would be more effective.

Exercise 2

1. Areas of need to consider for your assessment might include the following: mobility, sleep, family resource support, and patient's ability to cope with stress of injury.

2. In conducting an assessment of Andrea Wang it will be necessary for you to **know** the effects of a cord transection and the appropriate communication skills that will allow you to be supportive and gain the patient's trust. Your own **experience** with loss can also prove useful in anticipating how she is reacting to loss of function in her legs. Using **attitudes** of confidence and creativity can be useful. Your confidence will be displayed in showing the patient you understand her situation and will work with her closely in her care. Being creative in suggesting a family conference may yield very useful assessment data. **Standards** of ethics and the intellectual standard of complete assessment apply. Andrea Wang has the

ethical right to be informed and to choose to accept the family conference. A complete assessment of the patient's acceptance of her injury will improve the quality of the information you collect. Answers to the diagram are as follows: (1) b, (2) d, (3) e, (4) c, (5) g, (6) a, (7) f.

3. Here is some of the information you may have collected on Andrea:
   Sleep:
   Sleep interrupted by bright light, noise, and discomfort.
   States, "I sleep during the day, but deep down I feel exhausted and helpless."
   States. "I can feed myself now and move arms a bit but probably sleep less every day."
   Irritable when asked about bowel and bladder function.

   Support from family/friends:
   States, "Eric has been in, and he's very supportive. I just don't know what is going to happen."
   Family is normally close.
   States, "My family came in but everyone was so subdued, it just depressed me even more."
   States, "Other than Eric and my friends, there is no one who can take care of me. My parents need me to care for them. It overwhelms me sometimes."
   States that she has not talked much with family about injury; hopes this is not permanent.
   Note: Change-of-shift report notes that family does not come into room very much.

   Coping with stress of injury
   States, "I just don't know, I'm overwhelmed. I hope I will have some movement in my legs."
   States when asked to describe health, "Now I feel lost."
   Unable to toilet normally; limited movement likely prevents her from dressing and bathing herself.
   Admits to feeling depressed when family visited.
   Irritable/angry over incontinence.

4. Three nursing diagnoses and defining characteristics that apply to Andrea's situation include the following:

   a. Sleep pattern disturbance related to emotional stress of spinal cord injury
   Sleep is interrupted.
   Patient complains of not feeling rested.
   Her behavior has been irritable at times.

   b. Ineffective family coping: compromised, related to situational loss from Andrea Wang's injury
   Family withdraws from chance to be supportive.
   Patient expresses concern about family response during visit.

   c. Ineffective individual coping related to situational crisis of spinal cord injury
   Patient is unable to meet role expectations.
   She expresses hopelessness and fear.
   She cannot meet basic needs: toileting, feeding herself.

5. Andrea Wang's case is complex. The best answer is choice d. She is experiencing the problem of bowel incontinence because of the effects of spinal shock on normal defecation. Because of her paralysis, she is immobile and at risk for impaired skin integrity. The uncertainty of her prognosis, her unfamiliarity with her body and its associated changes, and the reaction of her family have caused great anxiety. The patient may also potentially have body image disturbance or self-esteem disturbance, depending on how she ultimately adjusts to the paralysis, but these diagnoses are premature. She is not in pain, her nutrition is good, and her condition is not chronic, therefore hopelessness is not applicable.

6. Goal: Skin remains intact without areas of breakdown through hospital stay.
   Outcomes: Skin is warm and dry, without areas of redness.
        Prescribed turning interval is achieved.
        There is absence of abnormal hyperemia.

7. To evaluate Andrea Wang's ineffective individual coping you can observe her verbal and nonverbal responses to discussions about her paralysis. Does she continue to express fear or depression? You can also evaluate the patient by observing her ability to begin problem solving and participate in rehabilitation.

Lesson 3 – Caring in the Practice Setting

Exercise 1

1. Comforting is conveyed not only through touch or the skillful performance of a procedure, but also by a neat, clean, and safe environment. Andrea Wang's room appeared neat and well-kept with no clutter from supplies or extra equipment. Her bed linen also appeared neat and clean.

2. The nurse establishes presence through the following behaviors:
   Using a calm tone of voice
   Acquiring the patient's consent
   Standing close to the patient's side
   Maintaining eye contact with the patient
   Presence conveys closeness and security. The nurse uses a calm and gentle tone of voice when he asks Andrea Wang if he can take her vital signs. By asking her consent, the nurse shows that he is open to her decision to make a choice. Standing close and using eye contact further conveys the nurse's experience and ability to care for the patient.

3. The nurse's behavior accomplished the following subdimensions of caring:
   "Doing For"   Comforting
           Performing skillfully
           Preserving dignity
   "Enabling"   Informing/explaining
           Validating/giving feedback
   The nurses' gentle, slow, and deliberate approach is comforting. He performs each assessment skillfully, being careful to compare findings on each side of the patient's body and moving methodically through all measurements. He preserves Andrea Wang's dignity by keeping her body well covered and draped during the examination. The nurse tells her which measurements he is taking and explains his movements to allay the patient's anxiety. He also gives feedback, saying "Good" several times to let her know she is doing well.

4. The nurse did not explain the purpose of various aspects of the examination. Adding simple and clear explanations such as, "I am going to check your abdomen to make sure you have good bowel function" would better accomplish the enabling subdimension of caring. By explaining the purpose of what you are doing, you keep the patient more fully informed. If Andrea Wang understands the purpose of the exam, she becomes less anxious with repeated assessments. More specific feedback concerning the nurse's findings would also be enabling and give the patient comfort through knowing her own clinical status.

5. The nurse asks the patient important questions.
   a. After Andrea Wang tells the nurse, "I can't believe this has happened to me," the nurse probes further and asks, "How does that make you feel?" This statement helps to assess the patient's feelings more thoroughly and centers the assessment on her feelings, not only on the injury.
   b. There are many opportunities to make this assessment even more thorough. For example, the nurse might ask, "Tell me what is most difficult for you at this time?" or "After

having such an active life, this type of injury must be frightening. Would you like to talk more about how you feel?" or "I know this injury makes you feel dependent. What does that mean to you?"

Exercise 2

1. The nurse displayed skillful technique, and she also anticipated. She expected Ira Bradley's response of feeling discomfort from the palpation of his lymph nodes. The nurse was able to anticipate, knowing that HIV infection involves the lymph nodes and that swollen nodes are usually painful.

2. There are several ways in which the nurse failed to show caring towards Ira Bradley. First, the nurse failed to listen. Had she listened more carefully, she would likely have rephrased questions. For example, she learned while assessing Ira Bradley that he had poor activity tolerance and was very tired. However she asked, "Has your tiredness interfered with you and your partner's sexual relations?" Ira's response was "What do you think?" The nurse might have instead asked, "Because you have been so tired, how has that affected you and your wife's sexual relations?" This response would have reflected listening and showed more compassion and understanding.

    The nurse also tends to exclude the wife by referring to her as "your partner." In addition, the nurse does not ask the wife questions directly to allow her to share her views, even though the wife does respond upon occasion. Finally, when Ira Bradley expresses his fears, the nurse does not explore them more fully when she has the opportunity.

    This case shows how a structured approach to assessment, although comprehensive, can sometimes limit the nurse's ability to truly know her patient and to show a sensitivity to his responses and concerns.

3. The correct answer is choice b. The greatest challenge for the nurse is to provide hope, because this patient has expressed numerous times his sense of hopelessness.

4. During the assessment of his values and beliefs, Ira Bradley says, "I value a day when I can get out of bed." One important approach to comforting is the control of symptoms. The nurse can realistically provide the patient options that might improve his symptoms enough for him to have a few quality days. For example, you already read in the nurses' notes that the patient had a better appetite on Wednesday. The nurse can build on that success to improve his calorie intake, which will give him more energy. The nurse can try comfort measures such as hygiene measures for his painful mouth and throat and sleep therapies to help him get necessary rest.

5. The correct answers are choices b and e. During the assessment of Ira Bradley's elimination status, the wife remarks, "There are a lot of changes. We don't know what to expect." This was an opportunity for the nurse to provide an explanation of symptoms and to allow the family to ask questions.

Exercise 3

1. The correct answer is choice d. The case manager's plan provides excellent recommendations for finding the family necessary resources to deal with their psychosocial and financial stressors. The plan offers support through enabling.

2. The clinical nurse specialist's plan focuses strongly on symptom control: controlling or minimizing infection, providing pain relief, and offering nutritional support. All of these approaches can provide Ira Bradley greater comfort and energy and help him to have a quality day when he can get out of bed.

Exercise 4

1. Both Andrea Wang and Ira Bradley are experiencing losses. Andrea Wang faces a loss in the ability to walk because of her paralysis. Ira Bradley faces a loss as a result of the change in his relationship with his wife and friends and by his impending death.

Lesson 4 – Physical Examination and Vital Signs

Exercise 1

1. The correct answer is choice a. *Tachypnea* is the term used to describe rapid respirations. The presence of a possible lung infection will impair Ms. Begay's oxygenation status and cause her to breathe more rapidly.

2. Crackles are sounds created by the sudden reinflation of groups of alveoli. They may be fine, medium, or coarse.

3. The correct answer is choice c. Auscultation with a stethoscope allows you to hear adventitious or abnormal breath sounds.

4. The correct answer are choices c and e. The nurse is using the appropriate size cuff. Sally Begay may sit during BP measurement, so her position is appropriate. The nurse did not palpate the brachial artery before cuff placement. The nurse also did not fully expose the arm as the gown sleeve was placed under the cuff. The bladder was positioned above the antecubital fossa, where the brachial artery is typically located. This nurse skipped important steps that could result in an inaccurate BP.

5. Sally Begay would benefit from a measurement of the patient's apical pulse. Fortunately, when you review the physical exam, you will find that the nurse does conduct this assessment.

6. Sally Begay's oxygen saturation reading is likely to be false because the nurse fails to remove the nail polish on her nail. The polish contains a pigment that can absorb light emission and falsely alter readings.

7. The correct answer is choice c. Extraocular movements are assessed by having Sally Begay follow the movement of the nurse's finger.

8. To measure extraocular movements correctly, the nurse must ensure that the patient keeps the head in a fixed position and faces the nurse throughout the entire portion of the examination.

9. Because Sally Begay may have an infection in the form of pneumonia, the nurse should be alert to note whether there is lymph node enlargement.

10. The nurse examines one carotid artery at a time to avoid possible occlusion of circulation to the brain.

11.

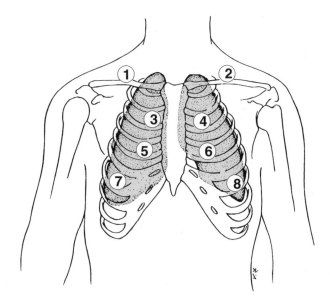

12. a. The nurse asked the patient to take a slow deep breath with the mouth open.
    b. The nurse listened to a full inspiration and expiration at each position of the stethoscope.
    c. The patient was sitting to allow for fuller chest expansion.

13. The correct answer is choice b. The nurse's exam would be more thorough if it included assessment for tactile fremitus. The possible accumulation of mucus in the airways from pneumonia would be detected from this palpation technique.

14. The correct answer is choice a. The patient's chest excursion can be reduced if pain is felt during coughing or deep breathing.

15.

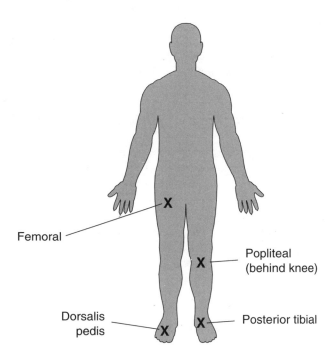

16. Both pulses are assessed together to determine equality and rule out presence of any factor that may obstruct blood flow to the lower leg.

17. Before conducting an examination of the abdomen, the nurse will collect a history that includes the following factors:
    a. History of abdominal pain—pattern may help nurse identify source during exam.
    b. History of recent weight change—will confirm any findings nurse may make regarding abnormalities of upper GI or lower colon.
    c. Patient's normal bowel habits—once nurse compares data with actual physical findings, a cause of elimination problem may be determined.
    d. History of alcohol ingestion—data may confirm findings of a liver problem during exam.

18. a. Yes
    b. Yes
    c. Normal bowel habits
    d. Yes

19. Use of an incentive spirometer will prevent atelectasis or further collapse of alveoli. This treatment will prevent development of pneumonia in the now uninvolved lobes of the lung. Upon auscultation of Sally Begay's lungs, the uninvolved left lung should remain clear with normal breath sounds.

20. Sally Begay has had pain during coughing. Pain may also occur during deep breathing. An analgesic will relieve that pain and help Sally Begay to breath more deeply during the treatment.

Exercise 2

1. Complete the report summary as completely as possible. If necessary, listen to the report a second time.
   Diagnosis(es): Head laceration, late-stage HIV
   Vital Signs: Stable; Temp 99.6; O_2 Sat 91%
   Mental status: When awake, alert and oriented to person and place
   Lungs/Oxygenation: Chest sounds clear; no cough; heart sounds normal
   Oropharynx: Dysphagia; oral intake better
   IV Site: Site in right forearm
   Lower Extremities: Good capillary refill; no swelling or warmth in calves; Homan's sign negative; extremities warm; all peripheral pulses palpable

2. Based upon information from the report, priority areas to examine are level of consciousness, oral cavity, lungs, and skin. Ira Bradley was admitted with a minor head injury. He also has HIV, which in its advanced stages can cause neurologic involvement. Follow-up measurement of level of consciousness will allow you to determine whether any changes are occurring. Ira Bradley has candidiasis, a yeast infection that has developed in his oral cavity. A thorough exam of the oral cavity is important to determine how the condition is progressing and whether the patient is responding to therapies. Because Ira Bradley has pneumonia, another complication of HIV, you will need to assess his lungs and thorax thoroughly. With the presence of an IV—and knowing that Ira Bradley has been dehydrated—an assessment of the skin will also be necessary.

3. Ira Bradley has HIV, a systemic infectious disease. Enlargement of the lymph nodes bilaterally confirms an active systemic infection.

4. The nurse's examination of the oral cavity was not very thorough. Your examination should include inspection of the inner oral mucosa and buccal mucosa. With the obvious presence of an infection, you need to determine how extensive the plaques are. Also look under the tongue and along the hard palate. A tongue blade will allow you to better visualize the posterior pharynx. Most important, because of Ira Bradley's diagnosis, if your examination is more thorough, you will need to wear gloves.

5.

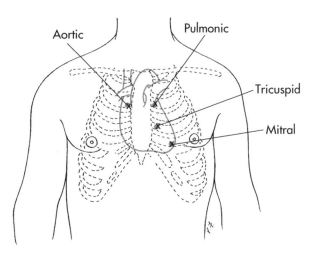

6. The correct answer is choice c. The nurse did not auscultate the second pulmonic area. In spite of the exclusion, she did auscultate methodically over the heart in order to detect abnormal heart sounds.

7. The correct answer is choice c. Tactile fremitus is measured to determine whether there is an accumulation of mucus or lung lesions in the lung tissue. With pneumocystic pneumonia, a common complication of HIV, and with the history of bibasilar rales, Ira Bradley is at risk for having congestion in the lung tissue and tactile fremitus.

8.

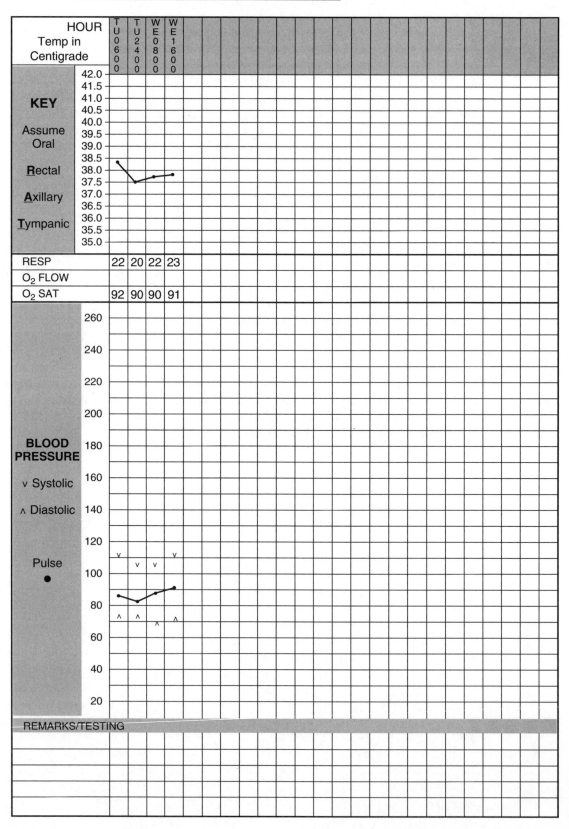

Vital Signs Record/
I/O and Parenteral Fluid Record

Date: _____

HOUR Temp in Centigrade	TU 0600	TU 2400	WE 0800	WE 1600												
RESP	22	20	22	23												
O₂ FLOW																
O₂ SAT	92	90	90	91												

KEY

Assume Oral

Rectal

Axillary

Tympanic

BLOOD PRESSURE

v Systolic

∧ Diastolic

Pulse
●

REMARKS/TESTING

9. Ira Bradley's heart rate could be slightly elevated for a variety of reasons: dehydration, anemia, and fever.

10. Ira Bradley's body temperature might have declined as a result of the 24-hour temperature cycle. Body temperature is usually near its lowest at around midnight.

Lesson 5 – Communication with the Patient and Health Care Team

Exercise 1

1. Because of Ira Bradley's diagnosis and the nurse's report describing Mrs. Bradley's concerns, it is likely you will face the possibility of both Mr. and Mrs. Bradley grieving. In addition, you should consider that when Ira Bradley was initially admitted, he suffered from some confusion. You will want to be alert for this since it can affect communication. Finally, the chart reveals a patient who has been ill for some time, suffers continuous exhaustion, and has few social supports. As a result, you also may face a situation in which the patient is depressed or saddened.

2. When the nurse enters the room to check Ira Bradley's vital signs, she demonstrates the following elements of professionalism:
     Courtesy
     Use of Name
     Privacy and confidentiality
   The nurse, Bentley, says "Hi" to Ira Bradley, introduces herself by name, explains her role as a nurse, and explains her purpose to check vital signs. The room has the privacy curtains pulled. Bentley uses good eye contact when first meeting the patient. She is also appropriate in asking his willingness to comply with having vital signs measured.

3. Bentley made the error of addressing Ira Bradley by his first name. It would have been more appropriate to address the patient in the following way, "Hello Mr. Bradley, my name is Bentley, I'm one of the nurses caring for you today. Do you prefer being called Mr. Bradley, or may I call you by your first name?"

4. During the interaction as the nurse assesses Ira Bradley's perception/self-concept, the patient uses good eye contact when talking with the nurse. He also uses a tone of voice that enforces his feeling of hopelessness. His facial expression further emphasizes his despair. Mrs. Bradley touches her husband's arm and sits close to his bedside.

5. It is important to understand the context of the nurse's interaction with Mr. and Mrs. Bradley. As a nurse, you will learn how each of these contextual factors influences your approach with the patient. In the case of Ira Bradley, several factors are interacting. The correct order of answers is as follows: e, a, a, b, c, a, b.

6. The correct answer is choice b. The nurse would be acknowledging the terrible stress and emotional burden that Ira's illness has created. Such an acknowledgement would encourage more verbalization. Choices a and c change the subject and do not focus on the true message the Bradleys are communicating. Choice d may have the intention of offering comfort to the patient but denies the source of Ira Bradley's stress and minimizes its enormity.

7. The correct answer is choice b. This question must be answered in the context of what you have learned about Ira Bradley. He initially tells the nurse that he does not feel comfortable discussing sexual issues. This signals a need for the nurse to be very sensitive. Information from the medical record revealed that he has been continuously exhausted. When the nurse asks about the effect of Ira Bradley's tiredness, it appears she has not been listening or attentive to his complete situation. Although fatigue is likely an issue, the nurse would have responded better by acknowledging that fatigue is likely making it difficult for the patient to have a good sexual relationship.

8. The correct order of answers is as follows: b, a, a, b, a. When the nurse asks closed-ended questions, the patient can simply answer with a yes or no response. Open-ended questions encourage more conversation and discussion.

9. The correct answer is choice d. Asking Ira Bradley whether he worked full- or part-time is posing a relevant question that will provide more detail about the patient's occupational history. It is not a clarification since the question does not verify the nurse's understanding of what Ira Bradley does. It is not an effort at focusing because the conversation has not been vague or rambling or unclear. The nurse's question does not summarize the patient's previous response.

10. The nurse responds to Ira Bradley's shrugging of the shoulders. She notes that he did not understand the initial question. She clarifies her response so that Ira Bradley is able to understand the question and provide a relevant response.

11. The following are examples of appropriate statements to make to the Bradleys.
    Sharing hope: "Mr. Bradley, you have shared that you value having a day when you can get out of bed. We will work with you to see if we can reduce your fatigue and improve your energy to the point that you can get out of bed more often and do more things for yourself."
       This response is not offering false reassurance. There are nursing approaches that can reduce Ira Bradley's fatigue and help to make his day more comfortable.
    Sharing empathy: "I think I understand how terribly difficult the experience of your illness has been for you and your family. It has affected all of you in so many ways. You have all tried to be so strong for one another."
       This response conveys the nurse's understanding of Mr. and Mrs. Bradley's feelings and reactions towards his illness.
    Summarizing: "A major factor in your illness has been the fatigue and exhaustion you feel. It has made it impossible for you to continue working, socializing with friends, and doing the things you enjoy with your family. Your illness has been unpredictable, causing you to have repeated infections. It is obvious that you are having difficulty remaining hopeful for what the future holds. I would like to help you discuss more your concerns about death and how you feel."
       This response summarizes some of the issues you were able to learn about Ira Bradley. A summary would then allow you to either focus on and clarify these issues or to define what he would like to reveal further.

Exercise 2

1. There are several interpersonal factors that may influence Sally Begay's communication. You would confirm all of these factors in your assessment when you meet Sally Begay:
   a. Trouble breathing
   b. Nausea
   c. The influence of her Navajo culture
   d. The close relationship she has with her family
   e. The fact that, according to her chart, she has a shy personality

2. When patients have difficulty breathing, they become short of breath and they tire easily during conversation. Their sentences are often shorter. They may not elaborate on open-ended questions.

3. The correct answers are choices a, c, and d. The report says that Sally Begay has stable vital signs, that she is going home today, and that she needs discharge teaching.

4. The nurse's introduction is very cursory. In fact she failed to introduce herself at all.
   Here is an example of a better approach: "Good morning, Sally Begay, my name is _____. I will be the student nurse caring for you today. I will be here until 3:00 p.m. It is time to take your vital signs—your blood pressure, temperature, heart rate. Vital signs help tell us how you are doing. Is it OK with you if I begin?"

5. The correct answer is choice a, an open-ended question.

6. In order to clarify Sally Begay's meaning about worries or concerns, the nurse might say, "Tell me more about what worries you at home."

7. The correct answer is choice c. The nurse could paraphrase the patient's response to send feedback that lets Sally Begay know how her message was understood—for example, "You say you will do OK at home, but your breathing and achiness are problems for you." However, confronting the patient therapeutically might provide a better response, particularly since you are preparing her for discharge today: "Ms. Begay, you say you will be able to care for yourself at home. However, you are also telling me that you tire easily and feel poorly. Will that not affect you?"

8. The correct answer is choice b. The conference is an example of communication in a social zone.

9. In the Admissions Profile you learned that Sally Begay relies on a medicine man. If the social worker and other health team members wish to improve the information communicated to Sally Begay, the involvement of the medicine man might prove helpful.

10. Here is an example of how you might terminate your relationship with Sally Begay: "Ms. Begay, I know you are going home today, and my shift ends this afternoon. I would like to summarize what we have done to help your breathing and give you a chance to ask questions about going home. The case manager has arranged a home health nurse to assist you when you get home, so you will have a good resource available."

Lesson 6 – Patient Education in Practice

Exercise 1

1. a. Carmen Gonzales has learning needs in the areas of managing her diabetes, which includes understanding her medications (insulin), diet, foot care, and exercise. She also has learning needs in regard to factors that influence her heart disease and how to manage the disease. She does not understand why she has foot infections, showing that her level of understanding of diabetes is likely poor. The fact that she has developed gangrene from repeated foot infections suggests she does not manage diabetes well.
   b. Patient has history of physical symptoms that may affect her ability to be attentive to teaching: pain and some difficulty breathing. She has also been very tired. As to her ability to follow any instructions, she reports there is nothing that interferes with her ability to follow advice or her medication schedule.
   c. Carmen Gonzales is reportedly pleasant and cooperative and has no known cognitive deficits. She prefers a translator to help her understand a discussion.

2. Her Physical & History reveals that she has received education in the past. She was instructed on diabetes mellitus and foot care 5 months ago. However the history also reveals that she does not know the names of her medications.

3. Her daughter, her husband, and the Spanish translator.

4. The best answer is choice d, lung congestion. A worsening of her congestive heart failure with developing lung congestion can result in shortness of breath or difficulty breathing. This symptom can become a significant barrier to a person's attentiveness to instruction.

5. The correct order of answers is as follows:
   a, c, d, g—Motivation to learn
   a, e—Ability to learn
   f—Resources for learning
   b—Learning needs

6. This question is a bit tricky. It appears that Carmen Gonzales has a need to learn valuing, a type of affective learning. She has perhaps not attached worth to the importance of eating correctly to control her diabetes. However, you would need to learn more from your patient, because the problem might also be comprehension or application, cognitive learning behaviors. The approach used to teach her 5 months ago might not have been suited to her learning needs, motivation, or ability to learn.

7. Diabetes education can be very extensive and involved. The types of topics a patient must learn involve all of the learning domains. The correct order of answers is as follows: c, b, b, c, a, c.

8. It is important not to jump to a diagnostic decision without having complete information. Your current assessment reveals the following defining characteristics.

Ineffective Health Maintenance	**Knowledge Deficit**
Demonstrates lack of knowledge about basic health practices	Verbalizes lack of knowledge
Reports of observed inability to to take responsibility for meeting basic health practices	
History of lack of health-seeking behavior	
Expressed interest in improving health behavior	

Carmen Gonzales has reported not knowing the names of her medications and denies having received instruction in the past. Her reported/observed inability to take responsibility for meeting basic health practices includes her not having a regular MD or having routine GYN checkups. Not having a regular MD also suggests she does not have health-seeking behavior. She did express willingness to work with the RN on a teaching plan.

9. The best diagnosis for Carmen Gonzales at this time is Ineffective health maintenance. Further assessment is actually needed to determine whether Knowledge deficit is an issue as well. You would need to determine what instruction was actually provided 5 months ago and then question the patient on her knowledge. For example, if she was instructed on her medications, you might assess what meds (insulin) she is currently taking for diabetes and what the medication is for.

10. Choice a is the correctly worded learning objective. It contains a singular behavior (identification of meal plan), an observable or measurable content (foods allowed within an 1800-calorie diet over a 24-hour period), and a timing condition (day of discharge).

11. Carmen Gonzales will require short and frequent teaching sessions because she tires easily and has had other symptoms such as shortness of breath and pain. It would be wise to plan a teaching session at least an hour or so after pain medication has been administered, to see whether she is then more responsive. Begin your plan early before she is discharged.

12. It would be appropriate to cover all of these topics in an education plan, but chances are you would lose Carmen Gonzales' attention and not help her achieve control of her blood sugar to reduce the repeated infections she is experiencing. The three priorities are development

of a meal plan within calorie restrictions; methods for performing routine foot care; and physiology of diabetes and how it affects her blood sugar. These choices are based on the knowledge that the Carmen Gonzales currently has a high, uncontrolled blood sugar and she does not eat the proper foods within a diabetic diet. Her repeated leg infections imply she does not know how to monitor or care for her feet. Talk with your instructor about these priorities. His or her views may differ. The greatest challenge among the three priorities is to teach her how to perform blood glucose monitoring because of her history of poor compliance.

13. When you developed a plan of care, you should have considered the following:
    a. Incorporating Carmen Gonzales' daughter and husband in any teaching sessions and having the daughter help play a role in supporting good diabetic care practices.
    b. Incorporating short and frequent teaching sessions following periods of fatigue or pain.
    c. Using demonstrations (perhaps food models) in your teaching.
    d. Incorporating the translator into the plan.
    e. Finding food types within Carmen Gonzales' preferences that can be included in a diabetic diet.

14. The best answer is choice c. Foot care can best be taught by showing Carmen Gonzales how to inspect and cleanse the feet through demonstration. A good time would be during her routine bath. However, as an adjunct, printed material might provide a way to show her the type of lesions or skin changes to look for.

15. In her health history, under Cognitive/Perceptual, she said she still saw things a little fuzzy. Typically, this is due to swelling of the lens caused by her diabetes being out of control.

16. The correct answer is choice c, discovery. This is an excellent way to teach Carmen Gonzales problem solving, specifically how to choose foods within her dietary preferences while still maintaining an 1800-calorie limit.

17. The correct order of answers is as follows: b, a, c.

Exercise 2

1. The correct answer is choice c. Psychosocial adaptation to illness is critical in considering how you will assess Andrea. You must anticipate that she is struggling to accept the impact of her injury. Whether she will be able to learn depends on her level of acceptance of what has happened to her.

2. The correct order of answers is as follows: b, d, a. Andrea shows bargaining by expressing a hope she will have some movement. Her anger is expressed in her unwillingness to discuss her incontinence. Her denial is expressed in not believing the accident has happened.

3. You should respond by explaining that because of Andrea's denial and anger, she is not prepared to learn about topics pertaining to her future. Going home is still quite a while away. She will require instruction that is in the present tense, dealing with issues she absolutely needs to know.

4. The best answer is choice c, discovery.

5. Group instruction is an option. You would have to acquire Andrea's approval, but she has stated that she considers her family to be close. Discovery can be used as well during group instruction so that Andrea and her family can do some problem solving. For example, what way works best for her to feed herself once she is sitting up? The family can learn how to assist her initially in setting up a meal.

Lesson 7 – Documentation Principles

Exercise 1

1. Complete the report form, including key assessment findings.

2. The nurse's report should lead you to the following order of actions to follow up and determine whether the patient's condition is stable or changing: e, d, a, c, b.

3. a. Check for depth of breathing, measure chest excursion: The nurse did not check excursion by palpating the chest. However, by checking the lung sounds, she did note symmetry of chest expansion.
   b. Inspect leg and trunk for condition of skin: The nurse's assessment was weak in this area. She briefly looked at the patient's legs, giving a bit more attention on the right side, where you might have noticed the discoloration from bruising and abrasion. She did not inspect extensively enough to determine size of abrasion, although she would have noted whether there was any drainage.
   c. Palpate pulses of upper and lower extremities: She palpated both upper and lower extremity pulses, finding them strong bilaterally.
   d. Inspect condition of IV in hand: On the video you could see the IV in David Ruskin's left hand. The nurse did not inspect condition of the IV.
   e. Ask patient to identify location of pain and rate intensity: The nurse asked the patient whether he had pain and if so, how intense it was. The patient reported chest pain at a level of a 7.

4. a. The nurse's change-of-shift report cited that the patient had "some pain in the left side and arm." It is likely that this is inaccurate, because the patient's injuries are all on the right side.
   b. As the nurse, you would still assess whether the patient had pain in the left arm and side. Then you would confer with the nurse who gave report to clarify her intent.

5. David Ruskin was admitted at 8:00 p.m., which is 2000 in military time. The first nurse's note was entered at 2030, or 8:30 p.m.

6. The note does not keep information about David Ruskin's right arm as organized as possible. Here is an example of a more organized note:
   "Patient admitted from Post Anesthesia Care Unit @ 2000. Awake, oriented to person, Glascow coma scale 15. Right arm elevated on sky hook, dressing is clean and intact, fingers of right hand have 1+ edema. Vital signs, color, and sensation all WDL."

7. a. The note was written at 4:15 p.m.
   b. The note is incomplete, because if the nurse assessed that David Ruskin's confusion was related to the pain medication, the nurse should have documented which pain medication was administered, as well as the patient's behavior after the medication was given. There is not enough information to support that the pain medication contributed to the patient's confusion.

8. In rewriting the note, remember D is for data, A is for action (or nursing intervention), and R is for patient response.
   D: During the last two assessments (0800 and 1200), the patient has stated, "My pain hasn't been nearly as bad today as it had been. My sides still hurt when I take a deep breath, but nothing like before."
   A: Continue PO med for pain and monitor as before. Pulmonary toilet q2h while awake. Teach and review chest splinting.
   R: Patient's pain has steadily decreased since transferring to our unit from 7 on Monday evening, down to a 3 today. Asked to rank pain. With pain medication, no more than 4. Respiratory rate 21 with some guarding.

9. The correct answers are choices b and d. As you review data on the assessment flow sheet there are elements that require the nurse's follow-up: status of edema and movement. Both reflect the condition of David Ruskin's right arm and hand. The nurse will track edema to determine whether it is increasing or decreasing, which reflects the patient's circulatory status. Movement should be assessed to determine whether pain is successfully controlled and whether movement thus improves.

10. Charting by exception.

Exercise 2

1. Completed flow chart:

Day/Time	Sat admit	Sat 2000	Sun 0800	Sun 1600	Sun 2400	Mon 0800	Mon 1600	Mon 2000	Mon 2400
Temp	100.2	100.3	100.8	100.4	99.8	100	101	100	99.6
BP	134/76	160/90	155/86	152/84	152/81	148/82	147/81	145/80	150/82
HR	98	110	100	100	98	96	104	104	90
RR	26	25	23	24	23	22	23	22	20
O$_2$ Sat		93%	93%	94%	93%	93%	94%	95%	94%
Pain		3	4	3	0	2	3	4	2

Admission diagnoses: Respiratory distress/FUO (fever of unknown origin)/pneumonia
          Sick to stomach

Significant past history: Myocardial infarction (heart attack) 5 years ago
          History of chronic bronchitis for 10 years

From the assessment data, identify four criteria to be concerned about, knowing Sally Begay has pneumonia:

        Respiratory pattern, lung fields, cough, and sputum

2. The correct order of answers is as follows: c, c, b, a, a, c.

3. The note does not identify where the chest pain is located (right or left), the quality of the pain (sharp or dull), or whether anything relieves the pain (e.g., positioning, splinting). The lung sounds are not described for the left side. In this example, the note is not complete.

4. Her oxygen saturation improves from 87% to 92%; however on Sunday the nurse notes that the oxygen saturation drops during exercise. The follow-up information in the record allows you to see the patient's response to therapy.

5. Identify the type of pain medication and the dosage that effectively helped Sally Begay breathe more easily.

6. **P:** Altered respiratory pattern; Impaired gas exchange; Altered nutrition: less than body requirements; Fatigue.
   I: Continuing to ambulate patient, up in chair 30 min. Oxygen at 2 l per nasal cannula. Continuing pulmonary toilet. Snacks offered when eating less than 50% of meal. Oral hygiene provided.
   E: Walked 30 feet, O_2 sat dropped to 89% on O_2. Coughing productively. Short of breath. States she feels tired after activities. Crackles heard in right middle and lower lobes. Left lung fields clear. Temp 99.6–100.2, RR 20–23. Ate 50% of meal, states no n/v but still not too hungry.

7. On the basis of information from the change-of-shift report:
   a. 87%
   b. Not reported
   c. Decreased
   d. The report was from the night shift. It would be unlikely that Sally Begay would receive a meal or snack during that time. The nurse reported that she slept.

Lesson 8 – Safe Medication Administration in Practice

Exercise 1

1. David Ruskin has no allergies.

2. The correct answer is choice b. Cefoxitin is a cephalosporin antibiotic administered to prevent development of infection from injury to soft tissues and bone.

3. 2100 is the time for his next scheduled dose.

4. a. The maximum dose of 10 mg can be given each time oxycodone is administered.
   b. The earliest he could receive another dose is in 4 hours.
   c. PRN means the medication is to be given when the patient requires it. A minimum interval of 4 hours is set for the time of administration. It cannot be given more often than every 4 hours.

5. Within the first 24 hours of his injury, David Ruskin's pain was quite severe, with pain ratings ranging between 8 and 7. Ketorolac is a potent analgesic NSAID with strength comparable to morphine. Typically, as a patient's pain is anticipated to decrease in severity, physicians change medications from IM to PO to give patients an analgesic not as strong and to avoid trauma from repeated injections.

6. $\dfrac{30 \text{ mg}}{15 \text{ mg}} \times 1 \text{ ml} = x$

   $\dfrac{2}{1} \times 1 \text{ ml} = 2 \text{ ml}$

7. The correct answer is choice a.

8. She checked David Ruskin's arm band against the Medication Administration Record.

9. She did not ask David Ruskin to state his name.

10. The correct order of answers is as follows: b, a, b, c, a, b.

11. The following changes would be expected:
    His pain acuity score falls.
    He grimaces less when sitting up.
    The pain along his rib cage decreases.

Exercise 2

1. The correct order of answers is as follows: d, e, c, a, b.

2. The correct answer is choice b. Furosemide will promote diuresis, thus reducing edema in the dependent extremities and intravascular fluid volume, which can cause pulmonary congestion. As a nurse, note that increasing edema and development of abnormal lung sounds can indicate a worsening of congestive heart failure.

3. The correct answer is choice d, allergic reaction.

4. Cefoxitin is the drug most likely to cause the reaction because it is an antibiotic. However almost any drug can cause an allergy.

5. The nurse checked each medication against the Medication Administration Record.

6. The correct answer is choice b. It generally takes 30 minutes for an oral medication to be absorbed and its action to take effect.

7. Both cefoxitin (IVPB) and insulin (SQ) can create rapid effects. Cefoxitin enters the blood stream directly and will cause the most rapid response.

8. Convert milligrams to grains before computing the necessary dosage.

9. The correct answer is choice a. Only regular insulin is used for a sliding scale. Insulin is always ordered in units. Use intrasite rotation to provide more consistency in drug absorption. Administer insulin subcutaneously at a 45- to 90-degree angle, depending on the patient's subcutaneous tissue.

Lesson 9 – Comfort

Exercise 1

1. A review of David Ruskin's Admissions Profile indicates he has experienced trauma in three areas. Each may be a source of discomfort.

Source	Location
Fractured right humerus	Pain likely along length of upper right arm from elbow to shoulder.
Laceration of scalp	Uncertain—Admissions Profile does not indicate location of laceration.
Abrasion	Uncertain—does not designate right or left calf/flank.

2. The description is poor. When describing pain location, use anatomic landmarks and descriptive terminology that specifically identify the source of pain. As for the abrasion, is the right or left calf involved? Where is the location of the laceration? How large is the laceration?

3. Because David Ruskin has experienced multiple injuries to the extremities and a laceration of the scalp, you might expect to see pain affecting the following areas:
Sleep
Mobility
Chest expansion
Respiratory pattern

4. Sympathetic stimulation resulting from pain typically causes the following physiologic reactions:
↑ Heart rate
↑ Respirations
↑ Blood pressure

5. David Ruskin's response indicated the following:
↑   Heart rate
no change Respirations
↑   Blood pressure

His heart rate was slightly elevated from baseline. This could have been due to the anxiety of being in the hospital as much as his pain. His blood pressure was significantly elevated for someone who reportedly has a normal BP of 110/60. An important factor to consider in David Ruskin's case is that he is a well-conditioned triathlete. His heart rate will normally be slower at rest. Pain is indeed causing an increase in vital signs, but the heart rate response might not be as great, because of his conditioning. *Study Tip: Review factors that influence heart rate in Chapter 31.*

6. The administration of analgesics for David Ruskin followed these principles:
a. Injectable medications (fentanyl and ketorolac) were administered initially to provide quick relief for David Ruskin's severe pain.
b. A milder analgesic was available for mild to moderate pain.
c. The ordered dosage of oxycodone was appropriately at the upper end of normal.

7. The analgesics were ordered PRN. David Ruskin was experiencing acute pain for almost 2 days, with pain ratings still at 7 throughout Monday. An around-the-clock (ATC) administration schedule is best, because it better ensures that analgesics are given before pain increases in severity. You no longer chase the pain; instead you control or minimize it.

8. The nurse wants to acquire a more detailed assessment of the condition of David Ruskin's injuries and to what extent they may affect his overall physical condition.
a. Head and neck: The nurse will inspect the condition of the scalp laceration, looking at the color of the skin (bruising?), presence of edema, depth and appearance of laceration, presence and character of any drainage. Palpation of the area around the laceration will determine whether there is local tenderness.
b. Chest and upper extremities: A priority is to examine the area of the fracture, which was surgically repaired. David Ruskin had an ORIF (open reduction and internal fixation). There should be a surgical incision present to inspect. Also the nurse will examine the extent to which movement of the right lower arm and hand is limited. The patient's chart indicated that in the ER he complained of rib pain. The nurse will assess how well the patient is able to breathe deeply.
c. Abdomen and lower extremities: The nurse will inspect the condition of the skin where it is reported David Ruskin has a "road rash."

9. Whenever a patient has had some form of head injury, there is concern about injury to the neck. The nurse assesses David Ruskin's range of motion in the neck and the presence of any pain on movement.

10. Chest excursion measures the ability of a patient to expand the lungs bilaterally and equally. If David Ruskin had rib pain, there may be a reduction in chest excursion.

11. The nurse did not indicate that she examined David Ruskin's surgical incision. The nurse also did not examine the flank or calf area, where the road rash was reportedly indicated.

12. David Ruskin displayed three nonverbal behaviors indicating his discomfort. He groans while sitting up, he moves very slowly, and he grits his teeth.

13. Data from the chart, EPR, and physical assessment provide information in the following categories:
    Onset and duration
    Location
    Intensity
    Pain pattern
    Relief measures
    The Emergency Department Report reveals the onset was immediately following the bike accident when the fracture and road burns occurred. The duration of pain has been continuous for 5 days. Pain is localized primarily in his arm, but he also complains of rib pain. The intensity of pain has ranged from a high of 7 (although it was possibly higher in the ER) to a 4. The pattern of pain has not been explored very well, although the nurse knows that activities such as sitting up in bed aggravate David Ruskin's discomfort. She also knows that he has no pain when he turns his neck. We do not know whether the patient has tried anything to relieve pain, however the analgesics have provided some relief. There are no apparent concomitant symptoms, although it is unclear whether this was assessed.

14. a. Under the category of Activity, David Ruskin seems to accept that his injury will prevent him from competing in the next triathlon. He also anticipates having trouble cooking and attending to some of the household chores at home.
    b. With regard to Perception/Self-Concept, he is concerned as to how quickly he can get back on his bike, which is associated with his wanting to compete again as a triathlete. The pain has surprised David Ruskin and it is making him feel immobilized.
    c. David Ruskin's ability to sleep has been altered as indicated in the Sleep-Rest category.
    d. Finally, the assessment of the Coping/Stress category reveals that the accident has "put him out of action" and David Ruskin worries about the effects on his academics and research.

15. a. In the case of David Ruskin, it would be useful to know more about how the African-American culture responds to pain. This may assist you in ensuring that the patient is able to express his pain and in identifying the type of pain relief strategies he would accept.
    b. Your knowledge of nonpharmacologic pain therapies will be very useful. David Ruskin continues to have pain, even though analgesics have reduced the intensity. Nonpharmacologic therapies may afford added relief.
    c. A knowledge of family caring will also be useful. David Ruskin obviously has a close relationship with his wife and friends. Your ability to include the wife in the plan of care and to have David Ruskin's friends provide support can improve your effectiveness.

16. The combination of relaxation and guided imagery would be a good choice for David Ruskin. He appears to be a cooperative patient who is interested in his health. He has achieved a level of relief that would allow him to learn the relaxation and guided imagery exercises. Distraction also may prove useful. The patient is obviously an active individual. Lying in bed for any extended period of time can be boring and very nonstimulating. Offer him books to read. He has requested a pamphlet on the type of surgery he has had and the nature of bone healing. Provide him with those pamphlets.

Exercise 2

1. Complete the worksheet based on data from the EPR.

2. Carmen Gonzales reported nausea and poor appetite. Her assessment flow sheet also reveals that she has been restless and irritable. Her uncontrolled diabetes could also have produced nausea.

3. a. T
   b. F
   c. F
   d. T

4. Carmen Gonzales was obviously having continuous acute pain. The administration of morphine by the intramuscular (IM) route is a problem. Although morphine is absorbed more quickly IM than by the oral route, intravenous administration would have been better to create a more constant therapeutic plasma level of the medication. This patient would likely have benefited more from patient-controlled analgesia.

5. The nurse in the video did not assess Carmen Gonzales pain. Instead he assessed the condition of her wound. An assessment of pain would include asking her whether the leg continued to be uncomfortable. What was the location of the pain in reference to the leg wound? Did the pain radiate out from the wound, either up or down the leg? Did the pain affect her ability to move her lower leg or foot? Did a certain type of positioning relieve the pain in any way? With gloves on, you might palpate around the wound margins to determine the level of tenderness.

6. Because Carmen Gonzales does not sleep well and because she is not active and unable to build much exercise tolerance, there is a good chance of fatigue increasing her pain perception. In addition, her anxiety over whether she will be able to walk will also increase the perception of pain.

7. Carmen Gonzales' Mexican culture is most likely to influence the meaning pain holds for her.

Lesson 10 – Oxygenation

Exercise 1

1. The correct answer is choice d. Pneumonia is an acute inflammatory process that begins in the alveoli of the lung.

2. The correct answer is choice b. Pneumonia will cause an alteration in diffusion. Inflammation of the alveolar capillary membrane will slow the rate of diffusion of respiratory gases

3. The correct answer is choice c. The accumulation of mucus in the bronchi can cause chronic airway obstruction. This increases resistance to air traveling through the airways, making it difficult to deliver necessary oxygen and remove carbon dioxide.

4. The correct order of answers is as follows: e, a, b, d, c.

5. The correct answer is choice b. The mucus created from an infectious, inflammatory process is likely to be green or yellow, with a foul odor. It can also be very thick and tenacious.

6. Sally Begay was not suffering severe hypoxia, because she did not have any neurologic signs such as restlessness, anxiety, disorientation, or reduced consciousness. However she had an oxygen saturation of 87% on room air. Normal is greater than 93%. In addition she had clinical signs of an increased heart rate and elevated blood pressure. She also reported dyspnea. However remember that the patient has an infectious process and her body temperature was 100.1° F, which could explain an elevated heart rate as well. She is clearly at risk for hypoxia, requiring close assessment and appropriate intervention.

7. Sally Begay has a history of congestive heart failure. With heart failure there can be a developing enlargement of the heart, causing a shift of the PMI to the left.

8. a. Digoxin is a cardiotonic ordered for Sally Begay's congestive heart failure. The drug strengthens myocardial contractility.
   b. Hydrochlorothiazide is a diuretic, which promotes diuresis, thus reducing circulating blood volume. A diuretic improves congestive heart failure and lowers blood pressure.
   c. Erythromycin is an antibiotic used to treat Sally Begay's pneumonia.

9. The light was used to help the nurse inspect the neck for jugular venous distention. When patients have a history of congestive heart failure, there is a chance the jugular vein is distended when the patient is sitting up, indicating ineffective cardiac contraction.

10. The correct answer is choice c. The Physical & History revealed crackles in the right middle and lower lobes. It would be important to pay particular attention to these areas to determine whether there has been a change; increased or decreased rales.

11. The nurse places the sensor over a nail that is covered in fingernail polish.

12. The correct answer is choice b. You would expect a false low reading because the polish would interfere or block transmission flight.

13. The correct answer is choice a. Pain associated with a myocardial infarction or heart attack typically radiates to the jaw and to the patient's shoulder and arm. Sally Begay has a history of myocardial infarction 5 years ago.

14. The correct answer is choice b. With anemia a patient has a decrease in oxygen-carrying capacity of the blood. There is less available hemoglobin to transport oxygen to the cells.

15. Measures to monitor closely for change in oxygenation include the following:
    Chest expansion (Does her chest pain ever affect her ventilation?)
    Lung fields (Does her lung congestion change?)
    Cough (Does she continue to cough up sputum and can you observe its character?)
    Sputum (what is the appearance of the sputum?)

16. The correct order of answers is as follows:
    (1) c—Pathophysiology
    (2) f—Environment
    (3) g—Culture in preventive health
    (4) j—Pathophysiology
    (5) d—Experience with previous patients
    (6) a—Accuracy
    (7) e—Lab standards
    (8) i—Depth
    (9) b—Discipline
    (10) h—Curiosity

17. Your best choice is Impaired gas exchange. Note that common defining characteristics apply to both diagnoses. However the nature of Sally Begay's pulmonary problems—pneumonia and bronchitis, coupled with her heart condition (CHF)—suggest more of an impaired gas exchange clinical picture. She does not have difficulty with ventilation, which is more characteristic of breathing pattern difficulties.

18. The best answer is choice c. Coughing techniques will help Sally Begay continue to remove secretions from her upper and lower airways. She does not require suctioning since she is able to cough up mucus and she is not suffering serious congestion. Incentive spirometry is not needed because the patient is able to breathe deeply without restriction. If she were to have trouble coughing up secretions, chest physiotherapy would become very beneficial.

19. Positioning and increased mobility are important ways to assist in promoting lung expansion and reducing pressure on the diaphragm during breathing. Getting a patient mobile helps to reduce the risk of stasis for pulmonary secretions.

20. Oxygen can cause a drying effect on the mucosa, and with the presence of a cannula in the nose, the patient may occasionally breath through the mouth. The nasal cannula fits around the patient's ears, and the prongs fit into the nares. Skin irritation and erosion can occur around the nose and ears.

21. Sally Begay's fluid intake is relatively low. The average adult's intake is about 2200 to 2700 ml per day, with oral intake averaging 1100 to 1400 ml. The patient could become dehydrated, which would make it very difficult for her to mobilize her pulmonary secretions. Consult with the MD about increasing her fluid intake.

22. The correct answer is choice b. Fluids are desirable for thinning and loosening secretions. Continuing an IV is not a problem, particularly if she remains nauseated and is having difficulty taking fluids. The risk of increasing fluids is an aggravation of her CHF.

Exercise 2

1. The correct answer is choice a. David Ruskin has suffered a traumatic injury that has caused contusions and rib pain. The rib pain reduces chest wall movement, thus potentially reducing ventilation.

2. The correct answer is choice d. Think about how your own breathing would be guarded with chest pain. You would not breath as deeply; thus the diaphragm would not descend as much and the anteriorposterior diameter of the chest will not increase as it normally should.

3. The correct answer is choice b. David Ruskin would benefit from an analgesic prior to any attempt to improve his ventilation. Analgesics can improve patients' ability to cough and breathe deeply.

4. The correct answer is choice a. By preventing hypoventilation, you reduce the patient's risk for developing atelectasis.

Exercise 3

1. The correct answer is choice c. The partial transection of Andrea Wang's thoracic spinal cord will damage nerves that innervate the intercostals muscles from T6 and above.

2. With injury to nerves innervating the intercostals, there is a risk for reduced chest expansion. If serious, there could be hypoventilation and an increased risk for atelectasis.

3. The assessment data reveal that her lung fields are clear but decreased in the bases. If hypoventilation occurs, it will usually be recognized first in the lower lobes.

Lesson 11 – Activity, Mobility, and Skin Integrity

Exercise 1

1. After reviewing Ira Bradley's chart and electronic record, you should assess the following data:

   Metabolic Changes
   Nutrition/appetite: has poor appetite, low body weight for height
   Infection: fever, pneumonia, candidiasis of mouth

   Respiratory Changes
   Lung fields: crackles bibasilar
   Respiratory pattern: has some labored and shallow breathing
   Oxygen-carrying capacity: anemia related to HIV

   Cardiovascular Changes
   Heart rate: normal and regular rate
   Activity tolerance: reports state of continuous exhaustion

   Musculoskeletal Changes
   Strength: weak motor response
   Muscle condition: presence of muscle wasting present
   Activity level: one-person assist with most activities

   Integument Changes
   Skin condition: skin tenting
   Mucosa: dry

   Gastrointestinal Changes
   Swallowing: difficulty swallowing, painful to swallow

   Comfort Level
   Sources of pain: always some pain, painful to swallow

2. The best answer is choice b. The environment within the home will not have a direct effect on tolerance. However if a person's environment poses risks or hazards, one's motivation to be active could be affected. Also, the environment is very significant if patients live in higher elevations because of the reduction in oxygen within the atmosphere.

3. The best answer is choice b. Activity intolerance is manifested by dyspnea, fatigue, chest pain, increase in heart rate that does not return to resting rate for several minutes, increased respirations, and reduced oxygen saturation.

4. With increased inactivity, further stasis or pooling of secretions could develop. This is complicated by the presence of pneumonia. With increased secretions his respirations could become more labored and rapid as well. Lung sounds would reveal crackles in additional lobes of the lung.

5. Ira Bradley has several predisposing factors for a pressure ulcer: diarrheal stools that he has had in the past, dry skin with poor turgor, malnutrition, anemia, infection, and cachexia.

6. The best answer is choice c. The nurse did not explore how Ira Bradley's feelings about HIV and his impending death affect his desire or ability to stay active.

7. His wife can provide social support, an important motivational factor. She has stayed by Ira Bradley's side and could be a partner in helping to improve his activity involvement.

8. The best answer is choice d. Passive range of motion does not require enough involvement on the part of Ira Bradley. He is capable of moving his own joints. Isotonic exercise might be too much at this time, although you would like to see him progress to walking. There is no data to show that he requires gait training, and gait training is not a type of exercise. Isometric exercise is ideal for Ira Bradley in an effort to increase his muscle mass, tone, and strength.

9. Immobility has the following physiologic effects:

   ↓—Wound healing
   ↑—Heart rate
   ↓—Urine output
   ↑—Respiratory rate
   ↓—Bowel sounds

10. a. Ira Bradley has pneumonia in addition to his general inactivity. Deep breathing helps to expand the lungs, which helps to reduce the risk for atelectasis and further secretions forming in the small airways.
    b. You have learned that Ira Bradley is depressed and angry. It will be very important to work with him, establish trust, and develop a schedule in which he can make decisions about the pace and level of activity he performs.
    c. It is important to determine more about Ira Bradley's range of motion, strength, and coordination that existed prior to hospitalization. You will want to establish a plan of exercise that is realistic so that he can be successful.

Exercise 2

1. The best answer is choice c. Transection of the spinal cord at T5 and T6 results in bilateral loss of voluntary motor control below that level of the spinal cord. Andrea Wang has paralysis of the lower extremities and loss of function of bowel and bladder.

2. The correct order of answers is as follows: d, b, c, e, c, b, a.

3. Andrea Wang's poor sleep quality is likely due to the constant nursing care she is receiving. She requires frequent positioning changes, even during the night. Until she becomes more stable, the nurses also conduct frequent assessments and attend to her physical needs regularly.

4. Support from Andrea Wang's parents and her boyfriend Eric will be essential to help her cope with her injury. As the nurse you will need to spend time with the parents and Eric to determine their level of understanding of Andrea Wang's injury and their commitment to helping Andrea. Ultimately you will want to involve them in her care. The patient's own understanding of her injury will also facilitate her coping.

5. The correct order of answers is as follows: (1) d, (2) g, (3) j, (4) k, (5) c, (6) e, (7) a, (8) b, (9) h, (10) f, (11) i

6. (1) Occipital bone
   (2) Scapula
   (3) Spinous process
   (4) Elbow
   (5) Iliac crest
   (6) Sacrum
   (7) Ischium
   (8) Achilles tendon
   (9) Heel
   (10) Sole

7. The areas least likely to be a problem for Andrea Wang include the elbow and occipital bone because she is able to move these body parts and still has sensation when pressure develops. She may still have sensation in the scapular area, which you should test, but because her positioning is limited, this area is still at risk.

8. It is, of course, difficult to assign a score without hands on involvement with a patient. However data from the health history and chart suggest the following:

Sensory perception 2 (Because of spinal cord transection, she has no sensation in lower extremities.)

Moisture 3 (Difficult to rank—the assessment data in the EPR record her skin as dry. However in the health history, Andrea Wang hints about stool incontinence.)

Activity 2 (She has been confined to bed first week of hospitalization. Now her assessment data reveal that nurses are getting her into wheel chair. She cannot bear weight.)

Mobility 2 (Because of her paralysis and because she has not yet had rehabilitation, her ability to move is limited. The ADL data flow sheet reveals that one person must assist in turning or log-rolling her.)

Nutrition 3 (Difficult to assess. The nurses' notes reveals that Andrea Wang is not eating well and has a reduced appetite. Until the injury her nutritional status had been very good. Her mood could further reduce her appetite, needs to be watched.)

Friction and shear 1–2 (Difficult to assess. She still has spasticity in the lower extremities. Needs assistance to turn. Unable to lift herself.)

9. Andrea Wang's total score ranges from 13 to 14. This is below 16, which is considered high risk for pressure ulcer development.

10. Examples of nursing diagnoses and defining characteristics that apply:
Impaired physical mobility related to neuromuscular impairment: limited ability to perform gross motor skills, difficulty turning, limited range of motion of lower spastic extremities.

Risk for impaired skin integrity related to reduced sensation and inability to change position voluntarily (Risk factors—see Braden scale).

Toileting, dressing, grooming self-care deficit related to neuromuscular impairment: inability to get to toilet or commode, inability to manipulate clothing for toileting or dressing.

Bowel incontinence related to loss of rectal sphincter control: constant dribbling of soft stool, inability to delay defecation.

Disturbed sleep pattern related to interruptions for therapeutics and grief over loss: verbal complaint of not feeling rested, awakening earlier than desired, dissatisfaction with sleep.

11. The nursing care plan for Andrea Wang generally contains appropriate types of outcomes and nursing interventions, but there are inaccuracies and in some cases lack of specificity. Critique comments are shown in bold-faced type.

Outcomes

Patient's range of motion improves. (**Be specific—identify the joints affected by immobility and the range of motion to improve (for example: dorsal flexion improves to 25 degrees, plantar flexion improves to 45 degrees.)**

Patient's skin remains intact, without abnormal reactive hyperemia over bony prominences. **This outcome is appropriate.**

Patient's lung fields remain clear. **You might wish to specify "all lung fields bilaterally" since Andrea Wang had reduced breath sounds in the bases.**

Interventions

Change patient's position regularly while awake; position on side, supine, opposite side with HOB elevated 30 to 40 degrees

Specify a turning schedule. Remember, an appropriate turning interval is: turning interval – hypoxia time = suggested interval. *(Study Tip: Read Fundamentals of Nursing in your textbook.)* **Also Andrea Wang should be placed in the 30-degree lateral position when turned on side. The head of bed should be kept below 30 degrees to prevent shearing forces.**

Apply egg crate mattress to patient's bed. **Andrea Wang requires a pressure-reducing surface. Generally, an egg crate provides comfort only. A low air-loss system or an air mattress would be more helpful.**

Clean and dry skin thoroughly following any episode of incontinence. **This is an appropriate intervention, but if Andrea Wang is incontinent of stool regularly, you might also choose to apply a skin barrier.**

Instruct patient on technique for controlled coughing; have patient deep breathe and cough every 1 to 2 hours while awake. **This intervention is appropriate.**

Maintain patient's fluid intake at 1000 ml daily. **Andrea Wang has no history of heart or renal disease. Her fluid intake should be at least 2000 ml daily.**

Assist patient in performing passive range-of-motion exercises to lower extremities 4 times a day. **This is an appropriate intervention. You might choose to specify the number of repetitions each time you exercise.**

Assist patient in performing passive range-of-motion exercises to upper extremities 4 times a day. **Andrea Wang is capable of moving her upper extremities voluntarily and should be on progressive active range-of-motion exercises.**

12. Interventions marked with an X would be appropriate in caring for Andrea Wang:
    Chest physiotherapy (Not necessary at this time—Andrea Wang does not have pulmonary congestion.)
    X   Elastic stockings
    Hand rolls (Not appropriate—Andrea Wang can move hands freely.)
    X   Ankle foot orthotic device
    X   Monitoring of lab data

13. The correct answer is choice b. Following bed rest, patients often have an increased heart rate and a decrease in pulse pressure. A drop in systolic blood pressure can occur when rising to an erect position, causing fainting. Note that Andrea Wang was a well-conditioned athlete and that her heart rate has been at 60 or below. Her risk for orthostatic hypotension is probably low.

14. When performing passive range-of-motion exercises, always place a cupped hand under the joint to support it. Support distal and proximal areas as well with the other hand.

15. The correct order of answers is as follows: d, c, a, b.

Lesson 12 – Elimination

Exercise 1

1. Carmen Gonzales' 24-hour I&O totals are as follows:
   Intake:
       Oral = 775 ml
       IV fluids = 480 ml
       Antibiotic fluid = 200 ml
       24-hour total intake = 1455 ml
   Output:
       Urine = 1650 ml
       Stool = none reported
       Total output = 1650 ml

2. Her urinary output for 24 hours is normal. (Normal output is about 1500 to 1600 ml daily.) Because her intake is less than output, on the basis of I&O alone, she could be at risk for dehydration.

3. The correct answer is choice d. Carmen Gonzales' history of congestive heart failure means that her heart is unable to pump as effectively as normal. An excess of fluid intravascularly increases burden on her heart. Having an intake moderately lower than output maintains her at a desired fluid balance level.

4. Her ingestion of 2 to 3 cups of coffee per day. Coffee contains caffeine, which promotes increased urine formation.

5. Her urinalysis findings are normal.

6. When a clean-voided specimen is obtained, the patient must cleanse the external genitalia. If cleansing is not thorough, bacteria may be flushed off the skin and into the urinary specimen.

7. The correct answer is choice b. Furosemide is a diuretic, which promotes increased urine formation.

8. The best time to give a diuretic is in the morning so that the patient can diurese during the day and not during the night, when trying to sleep.

9. The correct answer is choice c. Carmen Gonzales' record shows that she gets up during the night to urinate (nocturia) and she reports a high frequency of urination.

10. Glucose can cross the glomerular capillaries into Bowman's capsule in the renal nephron. A high concentration of glucose pulls water with it and results in polyuria because of the diuretic effect.

11. The correct answer is choice b. The ability to take in fluids has no influence on a patient's ability to void.

12. The correct order of answers is as follows: b, b, c, b, a.

13. Several factors might have influenced Carmen Gonzales' ability to defecate a normal stool. She was nauseated for 2 days, which likely resulted in decreased solid food intake. Her nausea also likely reduced her oral intake of fluids. Her report of feeling exhausted may suggest her activity was reduced.

14. The correct answer is choice d. Chronic use of laxative causes loss of the normal defecation reflex.

15. Foods high in fiber tend to promote normal, soft-formed stool. Carmen Gonzales' diet contains many low-fiber foods. The correct order of answers is as follows: a, a, b, a, b, a.

Exercise 2

1. All choices are correct. With a spinal cord transection and spinal shock, sensory impulses cannot travel from the bladder to the brain's micturition center in order for Andrea Wang to sense bladder fullness. The external urinary sphincters fail to function properly with loss of voluntary control of urination. The GI system is also affected by her injury. There is a temporary reduction in peristaltic contraction. Andrea Wang will also experience loss of rectal sphincter tone.

2. The correct answer is choice c. Andrea Wang had a urinary catheter inserted at the time of admission.

3. Andrea Wang has high thoracic damage to the spinal cord. There is the likely possibility that her micturition reflex pathway will still be intact, allowing urination to occur reflexively. The physician hopes she will be able to function with a reflex bladder.

4. The need for regular physical assessment for bladder distention.

5. The correct answer is chioce d. Once Andrea Wang's condition stabilizes, she still may not be able to void voluntarily. Use of a straight catheter over the long term will provide a means to empty the bladder regularly and avoid risks posed by an indwelling retention catheter.

6. Intermittent drainage of the bladder causes less infection than continuous drainage from an invasive, indwelling catheter.

7. The correct order of answers is as follows: c, d, a, b, e.

8. Check the drainage tubing for kinks. The tubing might have become positioned under the patient or it may have become kinked in the side rail. Check the tubing frequently to ensure a smooth, uninterrupted flow of urine.

9. Andrea Wang's 24-hour I&O totals for Wednesday are as follows:
   Intake:
       Oral = 2300 ml
       IV fluids = 0
   Output:
       Urine = 1700 ml
       Stool = 0
       Other = 0
   Net for 24 hours = + 600 ml

10. Below are several nursing actions that you could institute for Andrea Wang's well-being:

Nursing Measure	Rationale
1. Keep all bed clothing and linen dry.	Promotes comfort
2. Keep the door of patient's room closed; close the privacy curtains during care.	Lessens embarrassment by giving patient privacy
3. Be nonjudgmental and show a consistent caring approach.	Develops trust with patient
4. Control room odors when incontinence occurs by removing soiled linen and using air freshener as needed.	Promotes psychologic comfort

11. Andrea Wang presents a number of factors that can alter normal peristalsis. The correct order of answers is as follows: b, a, a, b.

12. Docusate sodium is a stool softener aimed at preventing development of constipation.

13. The best answer is choice d. Incontinence results in the exposure of the patient's skin to urine and/or feces, causing irritation to the skin and creating the risk for pressure ulcer formation. If any incidence of fecal incontinence is not addressed quickly, a female patient in particular could be exposed to spread of microorganisms to the urethra, resulting in an infection.

14. Perform a guiac test on the stool to determine the presence of blood. Continuous stress can cause an increase in stomach acid secretion. A patient with spinal cord damage is at risk for a stress ulcer. Andrea Wang is receiving famotidine to reduce that risk.

Lesson 13 – Loss and Grief and Nursing Interventions to Support Coping

Exercise 1

1. The correct answer is choice c. The partial transection of the spinal cord with resultant paralysis is best described as an actual loss.

2. Andrea Wang's injury can pose other associated losses: loss of role as a student, loss of sexuality because of her relationship with Eric, loss of role as daughter and support person to her parents, and loss of dignity and self-worth.

3. The answer is no. Although there are stages of grieving well defined by several theorists, loss and the grief response are unique to each person. There is no timeline you can use as a nurse to know what stage of grief a patient is experiencing. Instead you must assess each patient's behaviors and emotions to determine the stage of grief.

4. Nonverbal responses displayed by Andrea Wang include the following:
Tone of voice—She expresses her frustration and anger when asked whether she would be willing to learn about changes in her bowel function.
Eye contact—She closes her eyes when expressing her frustration and helplessness. Specifically, she closes her eyes and looks away when asked about her perception of stress.
Gesture—She shakes her head several times when expressing her helplessness. When asked about her perception of rest, she sighs and shakes her head.

5. Andrea Wang reported difficulty sleeping. She is reported to have a reduced appetite, and she admits to feeling exhausted.

6. Andrea Wang expressed hopefulness several times during the interview with the nurse. She discussed the desire to go back to school eventually. She hopes to get back some function movement. She and her family are hoping the paralysis is not permanent. Finally, her ultimate hope is to be able to walk again.

7. Critical thinking will allow you to conduct a more thorough and meaningful assessment of Andrea Wang's needs. The correct order of answers is as follows: (1) d; (2) g; (3) i; (4) c; (5) h; (6) a (promotes autonomy); (7) f (preserves dignity); (8) b (demonstrates humility); (9) e (demonstrates creativity).

8. The best answer is choice d. This approach is less likely to put the parents on the defensive. It also keeps things present-oriented.

9. Examples of questions you might pose for Eric:
   "I know you are an important resource for Andrea. What concerns do you have about your relationship?"
   "What contributions would you like to make in helping Andrea with her rehab?"
   "Andrea's injury has been a terrible loss for her. What type of loss are you feeling?"
   "What will be most difficult for you if you choose to help Andrea?"

10. The best answer is choice b, intellectual indicator. We are not sure of the extent to which Andrea Wang is able to acquire new knowledge or skills. We do know her level of denial affects the type of information to present. The nurse's assessment has not really tested the patient's ability to retain information, stay attentive, etc.

11. The following defining characteristics apply:

Ineffective individual coping	**Hopelessness**
Sleep disturbance	Verbal cues (e.g., sighing; saying, I feel so helpless.")
Decreased use of social support	Closing eyes
Use of coping mechanisms that impede adaptive behavior	Decreased appetite
Fatigue	Increased/decreased sleep
Verbalization of inability to cope	
Inability to meet basic needs	
Inability to meet role expectations	

Both diagnoses are potentially applicable to Andrea Wang's situation and very closely related. However the patient has expressed hope (perhaps somewhat unrealistically), and she shows an interest in working with the health team on a rehab plan. Therefore, Ineffective individual coping might be the best diagnosis on which to focus nursing interventions at this point.

12. Additional nursing diagnoses that might apply to Andrea Wang's case include:
   Self-care deficit (bathing/hygiene, grooming, toileting)
   Impaired physical mobility
   Risk for impaired skin integrity
   Compromised family coping
   Disturbed sensory perception (tactile, kinesthetic)
   Ineffective sexual patterns

13. In developing your nursing plan of care for Ineffective individual coping, you should have considered the following:

Realistic involvement of family and Eric in the plan.

Use of therapeutic communication techniques in helping Andrea Wang express her fears and concerns.

Incorporation of the patient's coping resources (i.e. "I like to talk things through"; demonstrations).

Stress reduction interventions (i.e., rest, nutrition, access to additional resource such as the social worker).

Nursing interventions in relation to support of the grief process.

14. Answers will vary based on each student's perceptions.

Exercise 2

1. The correct answer is choice a—increased heart rate, part of the general adaptation syndrome.

2. The correct order of answers is as follows: c, a, b, b.

3. The correct answer is choice b. David Ruskin is already talking about the future. He has accepted his injury relatively well, although he does have concerns about his academics and his job in the lab. He wants to read about his injury so that he can be informed.

4. David Ruskin has experienced a temporary loss of function of his arm, in contrast to Andrea Wang's permanent injury. He does face role changes (student, work), but again, they are temporary. He reports that his relationship with his wife is very supportive, and he already acknowledges the effects the injury will have.

Exercise 3

1. a. Ira Bradley is experiencing the potential loss of life, which in this case is perceived because of the nature of his illness.
   b. He displays behaviors that seem to match Kübler-Ross's stage of depression. He realizes his disease is terminal and he feels overwhelming hopelessness.
   c. His social support consists primarily of his wife. The disappearance of friends makes Ira Bradley's illness difficult for both him and his wife. His wife is at his side and defends their relationship several times during the history. Her nonverbal responses to Ira Bradley's comments shows that she is experiencing a great deal of stress as well.
   d. Spiritual beliefs: Ira Bradley comes from the Jewish faith. This may become a resource as he begins to face his death.
   e. Loss of personal life goals: This is a significant issue for Ira Bradley. He at one time participated in a highly intellectual and technically skilled occupation. Now he is unable to work regularly. He faces loss of his sexuality and intimacy with his wife. At times, he feels very ill and exhausted and probably has difficulty interacting actively with his children.
   f. The family's grief is observed by watching the wife carefully during the interview. Mrs. Bradley frequently looks away as Ira Bradley discusses death openly. She might not be as accepting of the inevitable course of AIDS as is her husband. Her relationship with her husband has changed dramatically. She quickly tries to make the point that she and her husband are still able to cuddle and that they try to maintain a sexual relationship. But he explains that they do not have sex very often. Mrs. Bradley's role in the family has changed; she must now care for Ira Bradley, maintain her job, and support her children.

2. Examples of questions you might ask Mrs. Bradley:
   a. "You have said that some weeks are like old times, others are like hell. Tell me what those difficult weeks are like for you."
   b. "Your husband speaks about his death openly. How do you feel when he speaks of his death?"
   c. "Tell me how your husband's illness has changed things for you at home."
   d. "What are your beliefs about death?"
   e. "What fears and concerns do you have, knowing Ira Bradley's illness is terminal?"

3. Ira Bradley has numerous nursing care problems. Measures to promote comfort are an important part of his plan of care. Answers are as follows:
   e, f—Fatigue
   c, d—Pain
   a—Hydration
   b, c, g—Appetite

4. The best answer is choice b—listen attentively and offer empathy. Ira Bradley's depression often results in confusion, feelings of loneliness, indecision. Providing a presence and understanding his situation helps in moving toward acceptance of a loss.

5. The best answer is choice d—assisting in verbalizing and discussing future plans.

Lesson 14 – Self-Concept

Exercise 1

1. Your data is still limited because you have not yet met Andrea Wang. However, preliminary data suggest that body image will be influenced by the paralysis and the associated incontinence she is experiencing. Her roles—as a student, a child of her parents, and the girlfriend of Eric—may change significantly. Because you have not talked with her, it is not clear how her self-esteem is affected, but she states that she is unsure about her relationship with Eric (sexuality concerns). Her identity is at least temporarily changed because you know that paralysis makes her more dependent. She is capable of only partial self-care.

2. As you listen to Andrea Wang's health history, you should assess the following information:

   Identity
   Relationship with parents may change—she has taken care of them.
   Relationship with friends will change—may not participate in sports; typically goes out frequently with group of friends.
   "I don't know what's going to happen to them or me" suggests she is uncertain about the consistency she has known as a person.

   Body image
   Andrea Wang is having much difficulty accepting the incontinence that has developed from spinal shock.
   She hopes "to get function back and can't imagine being in a wheelchair." She wants to be able to get around again.
   Ability to care for herself is now limited—she can partially feed herself.

   Self-esteem
   Andrea Wang's ideal was to be an active athlete, a successful student in forestry, and a young woman with a steady relationship with Eric. It would appear she is well liked; she presents herself as a very likable person.
   Her injury threatens all of this.
   She sees herself right now as being dependent. She is depressed and overwhelmed.

Role performance
> Andrea Wang is concerned about getting behind in school.
> She normally helps care for her parents; now she does not know what will happen to them.
> Paralysis can influence how she has an intimate relationship with Eric.

3. The best answer is choice c. Self-concept is a combination of variables (identity, body image, self-esteem, and role performance) that provides a sense of wholeness.

4. The best answer is choice a. Andrea Wang's situation currently best reflects role overload. She has multiple roles—daughter, student, girlfriend—that are currently unmanageable because of the changes imposed by her injury.

5. The correct answer is choice c. Andrea Wang is showing some anger, especially in regards to incontinence.

6. As the nurse caring for Andrea Wang, you can present an accepting view (verbally and non-verbally) when she talks about incontinence or when you are required to provide needed hygiene. Do not avoid going into the room to talk with Andrea Wang. Her family seems to be doing this. Be very open to discussing her feelings about the paralysis. Give her time to vent her fears and concerns.

7. Choice d is correct. Her family may be close, but it typically is not her primary resource for problem solving. She may indeed think through issues with Eric and friends, but she clearly prefers to be the one to think through problems on her own. Spiritual or religious guidance seems unlikely to be helpful.

8. The correct order of answers is as follows: (1) b; (2) d; (3) c; (4) a; (5) e (creativity); (6) f (perseverance).

9. The correct order of answers is as follows: c, d, b, a, e. Andrea Wang's behaviors match the defining characteristics necessary to develop the nursing diagnosis of ineffective individual coping.

10. The following is an example of a nursing care plan applicable to Andrea Wang's case:

Nursing Diagnosis: Ineffective individual coping

Goal	Expected Outcomes
Will acquire support system within 2 weeks	Will discuss illness openly with parents and boyfriend in 3 days Will participate in group sessions involving other patients with spinal cord injury in 2 weeks
Will understand implications of spinal cord injury within 2 weeks	Is able to describe the effects paralysis will have on her bodily function Will be able to discuss potential complications requiring ongoing self-management Will identify goals to achieve within limits of injury

Interventions	Rationale
1. Set up family conference and have primary nurse and case manager attend.	Coping with devastating injury takes time and requires patient to use available resources.
2. Show interest in and accept patient's feelings and thoughts.	Supports patient in accepting own feelings.
3. Once patient asks more questions about implications of injury, refer her to a support group composed of patients who have experienced spinal cord injury.	Persons who have experienced similar illness can be very supportive.
4. Have nurse specialist conduct sessions explaining nature of spinal cord injury and its effects on bodily function.	Allows patient to establish a realistic view of what spinal cord injury involves.
5. Offer access to teaching resources such as pamphlets and videos.	Access to information supports patient's normal coping resource for problem solving.
6. Assist patient to conduct simple problem solving with limitations in self-care.	Problem solving reinforces coping resources patient already uses.

Evaluation

Sit in on family conference as a facilitator and observe patient's interaction.

During teaching session, have patient explain how spinal cord injury affects her normal function.

Ask patient to write a list of goals she wishes to achieve in the next 2 weeks of rehab.

Exercise 2

1. Ira Bradley's Admissions Profile reveals a number of factors that can influence his self-concept:

   b—Receives treatment for depression (An emotional deficit prevents him from assuming role as father and spouse.)

   c, d—Needs assistance with ADL (Dependency on others is a stressor to both self-esteem and identity.)

   c, d—Senses change in masculinity (Sexuality concern is a stressor to both self-esteem and identity.)

   a—Has late-stage HIV (Debilitating, terminal condition influences body image.)

   a—Is fearful of a painful death (Symptoms associated with advanced HIV influence body image.)

2. Several of Ira Bradley's behaviors reflect an alteration in self-concept:

   Shows anger

   Passive attitude

   Puts himself down

   (Note: The patient's long hair does not imply he has a unkempt appearance.)

3. Mrs. Bradley has considerable stress: her husband's illness and increasing dependency, her role as a mother, concern about the future, loss of social contacts. She is by her husband's side and attempts to minimize some of his concerns by reinforcing the positives. For example, she quickly insists that they still have some intimacy (cuddling). To maintain her family, she has tried to preserve Friday evenings together watching movies. She is interested in learning about her husband's condition and ways to prevent infection. She shows evidence of potentially good coping behaviors.

4. a. Confidence can be important when a patient suffers such a serious disease and has multiple health problems. You can show confidence in your approach to assessment by becoming familiar with HIV and directing questions that reflect your knowledge. You can also show Ira Bradley your confidence in your ability by sharing information that pertains to his illness. The confidence you show in communicating openly and empathically can also prove useful.

    b. Risk taking applies if you explore the patient's feelings about death more thoroughly. This can be difficult if you are inexperienced, either personally or in your experiences with patients. Ira Bradley speaks of his death often and needs to be able to discuss it.

5. Additional stressors include the following:

    Body image—He continues to suffer physical changes from his disease, including oral infection and muscle wasting.

    Role—Ira Bradley and his wife were part of their friends' social circles. Their roles as members of those groups have changed. In addition, Ira Bradley's role in his own family is threatened because his children have difficulty accepting changes related to his illness.

    Self-esteem—Financial instability resulting from Ira Bradley's inability to maintain part time job and his wife's threatened job security.

    Identity—The negative attitudes that friends have displayed towards Ira Bradley and his children add considerable stress to his identity as a human being.

6. The correct answer is choice c. Middle-age adults begin to reflect and reevaluate whether they are satisfied with what they have accomplished. This gives them the chance to change directions.

7. Teaching approaches:

    Determine how well Ira Bradley can physically tolerate instructional sessions and plan short teaching sessions.

    Include his wife and when appropriate, his children, in teaching sessions.

    Focus education on those aspects of Ira Bradley's disease that can be managed.